# CANCER TREATMENT UPDATES: JANUARY 2024 – OCTOBER 2024

Kerry Atkinson

**About this book**

The painting on the front cover "Whale Beach – Luminous Dawn" was painted by the author.  All the text was written by the author.

**Key words**

Cancer; cancer treatments update; 2024

**Other books by Kerry Atkinson**

**Medical books**

1. Graft-versus-Host Disease. Editors, S Burakoff, H J Deeg, J Ferrara, K Atkinson. Marcel Dekker Inc, New York, 1990.
2. Clinical Bone Marrow Transplantation. First edition. Editor, K Atkinson. Cambridge University Press, Cambridge UK, 1994.
3. The BMT Data Book: A Manual for Bone Marrow and Blood Stem Cell Transplantation. K. Atkinson, Cambridge University Press, Cambridge UK, 1998.

4. Clinical Bone Marrow and Blood Stem Cell Transplantation. Second Edition. Editor, K. Atkinson. Cambridge University Press, Cambridge UK, 2000.

5. Clinical Bone Marrow and Blood Stem Cell Transplantation. Third Edition. Eds, K. Atkinson, R Champlin, J Ritz, M Brenner, P Ljungman and W Fibbe. Cambridge University Press, Cambridge UK, 2004.

6. The BMT Data Book. Second edition. R Munker, HM Lazarus and K. Atkinson, Cambridge University Press, Cambridge UK, 2009.

7. The BMT Data Book: Including Cellular Therapy. Third edition. R Munker, C Hildebrandt, HM Lazarus and K. Atkinson, Cambridge University Press, Cambridge UK. 2013.

8. Hematopoietic Cell Transplants: Concepts, Controversies and Future Directions. Eds HM Lazarus, RP Gale, A Keating, A Bacigalupo, R Munker, K Atkinson, A Syed. Cambridge University Press, Cambridge, UK. 2017.

9. The Biology and Therapeutic Application of Mesenchymal Cells. Ed. K Atkinson. Wiley/Blackwell. 2017

10. Revolutionizing Tropical Medicine. Eds. K Atkinson and D Mabey. Wiley/Blackwell Publishers Inc. 2019.

11. Asthma: Targeted Biological Treatments 2020. Kindle Direct Publishing, 2020. e-book and paperback

12. Atopic Dermatitis: Targeted Biological Treatments 2020. Kindle Direct Publishing, 2020. e-book and paperback

13. Psoriasis: Targeted Biological Treatments 2020. Kindle Direct Publishing, 2020. e-book and paperback

14. Crohn's disease and ulcerative colitis: Targeted Biological Treatments 2020. Kindle Direct Publishing, 2020. e-book and paperback

15. Rheumatoid arthritis, Juvenile Idiopathic Arthritis, Ankylosing spondylitis, Psoriatic Arthritis and Gout: Targeted Biological Treatments 2020. Kindle Direct Publishing, 2020. e-book and paperback

16. Small Cell Lung Cancer: Targeted Biological Treatments 2020. Kindle Direct Publishing, 2020. e-book and paperback

17. Chronic Myeloid Leukemia: Targeted Biological Treatments 2020. Kindle Direct Publishing, 2020. e-book and paperback

18. Melanoma: Targeted Biological Treatments 2020, Kindle Direct Publishing 2020. e-book and paperback

19. Dementia - A Caregiver's Guide. Kindle Direct Publishing 2020. e-book

20. Breast Cancer: Targeted Biological Treatments 2021. Kindle Direct Publishing 2021. e-book and paperback

21. Non-melanoma Skin Cancers: Targeted Biological and Specifically Designed Therapeutic agents. 2022. Kindle Direct Publishing 2021. e-book and paperback

22. Hodgkin Lymphoma: Targeted Biological Treatments. 2022. Kindle Direct Publishing 2022. e-book and paperback

23. Chimeric Antigen Receptor (CAR) T Cells: The second Revolution in Cellular Therapy. 2022. Kindle Direct Publishing 2022. e-book and paperback

24. Acute lymphoblastic leukemia: targeted immune therapeutic agents. Kindle Direct Publishing 2023. e-book and paperback

25. Artificial Intelligence and Medicine. A book in the Modern Medicine series. Kindle Direct Publishing 2024. e-book and paperback

26. Artificial intelligence in medicine. Volume 2: Clinical applications before the availability of CHAT-GPT4. Kindle Direct Publishing 2024. e-book and paperback

27. Non-small cell lung cancer: new inhibitory designer drugs approved for its treatment. Kindle Direct Publishing 2024. e-book and paperback

**Natural history/conservation books**

28. Bird facts for everyone. K Atkinson. Outskirts Press Inc., Denver, USA. 2014

29. Birds, Birds, Birds. Kindle Direct Publishing 2020. e-book and paperback

30. A Field Guide to the Wild Habitats of Sydney Australia. Kindle Direct Publishing 2021. e-book and paperback

31. Conserving New Zealand's Endangered Species. Kindle Direct Publishing 2021. e-book and paperback

32. Conserving Australia's Endangered Species. Kindle Direct Publishing 2021. e-book and paperback

33. Nature's Wonders: Britain and Ireland. Kindle Direct Publishing 2021. e-book and paperback.

34. Nature's Wonders: Spain and Bulgaria. Kindle Direct Publishing 2022. e-book and paperback.

35. Nature's Wonders: France's Camargue, the Swiss National Park and Portugal. Kindle Direct Publishing 2022. e-book and paperback.

36. Nature's Wonders: Cuba. Kindle Direct Publishing 2022. e-book and paperback.

37. Nature's Wonders: Japan in Winter Kindle Direct Publishing 2022. e-book and paperback.

38. Nature's Wonders: India. Kindle Direct Publishing 2022. e-book and paperback.

39. Nature's Wonders: Tanzania. Kindle Direct Publishing 2022. e-book and paperback.

40. The Silk Road: Uzbekistan and Kazakhstan – A Book in the Nature's Wonders Series. 2022. Kindle Direct Publishing 2022. e-book and paperback.

41. Madagascar – Land of Lemurs and Chameleons: a book in the Nature's Wonders series 2023. Kindle Direct Publishing 2022. e-book and paperback.

42. South Africa - Kalahari to the Cape - a book in the Nature's Wonders series. Kindle Direct Publishing 2022. e-book and paperback

43. Nature's Wonders – Finland - land of owls and lakes. Kindle Direct Publishing 2023. e-book and paperback

44. Nature's Wonders – Ethiopia. Kindle Direct Publishing 2023. e-book and paperback

45. Nature's Wonders – Kakadu National Park and Central Australia. Kindle Direct Publishing 2023. e-book and paperback

46. Nature's Wonders – Lord Howe Island, Australia. Kindle Direct Publishing 2023. e-book and paperback

47. Norway above the Arctic Circle in March. A book in the Nature's Wonders series. Kindle Direct Publishing 2024. e-book and paperback

48. The Inside Passage and the Pribilof Islands. A book in the Nature's Wonders series. Kindle Direct Publishing 2024. e-book and paperback

49. Orca! (and some interesting bird species in Washington State). Kindle Direct Publishing 2024. e-book

50. Big game and big fish. A book in the Nature's wonders series. Kindle Direct Publishing 2024. e-book and paperback

**Other books**

51. Paintings by Kerry Atkinson 2019 – 2021. Kindle Direct Publishing 2021. e-book and paperback.

52. Ferrari Road Cars. Kindle Direct Publishing 2022. e-book and paperback.

53. Paintings by Kerry Atkinson. 2022. Kindle Direct Publishing 2022. e-book and paperback.

54. Samuel Beckett and Bob Dylan – living in a Shakespearean era. Kindle Direct Publishing 2022. e-book and paperback.

55. Paintings and sculptures by Kerry Atkinson. 2023. Kindle Direct Publishing 2023. e-book and paperback.

56. Ten influential European paintings. Kindle Direct Publishing 2023. e-book and paperback

57. The Pillars of Rock 'N Roll. Kindle Direct Publishing 2024. e-book and paperback

58. Buildings as sculptures. Kindle Direct Publishing 2024. e-book and paperback

**"Then you better start swimmin' or you'll sink like a stone**
**For the times they are a-changin'"**

From Bob Dylan's song "The times they are a-changin" from his album "The times they are a-changin" released by CBS Records in 1964

## TABLE OF CONTENTS

## Author's preface

Like many areas of human activity, medicine is developing very rapidly. This is due to the recent approval of many new drugs, gene therapies and cell therapies. These new discoveries have resulted from the comprehensive understanding of the biology of both normal human cells and abnormal human cells. This tsunami of new therapeutic products is changing treatment algorithms. Oncology has benefited more than any other speciality from these new therapeutic products.

This book describes these new advances in cancer medicine.

- *Chemotherapy de-escalation using an 18F-FDG-PET-based pathological response-adapted strategy in patients with HER2-positive early breast cancer (PHERGain): a multicentre, randomised, open-label, non-comparative, phase 2 trial*[12]

The 3-year follow-up of this trial suggests that early noninvasive imaging might identify patients who can be treated with trastuzumab and pertuzumab.

The PHERGain trial is a recent example of using early signals provided by $^{18}$fluorine-fluorodeoxyglucose positron emission tomography ($^{18}$F-FDG-PET) to determine therapy.

Patients with HER2-positive invasive breast cancer (stages I–IIIa) were randomized in a 1:4 ratio to:

1. Standard docetaxel, carboplatin, trastuzumab, and pertuzumab (TCHP) (Group A)

or

2. Trastuzumab and pertuzumab without cytotoxic chemotherapy (Group B)

71 and 285 patients, respectively, were randomized

Patients underwent surgery, received endocrine therapy if appropriate, and received HER2-directed therapy postoperatively. They received $^{18}$F-FDG-PET scans at baseline and after 2 cycles of neoadjuvant therapy. Patients in group B who showed response using $^{18}$F-FDG-PET scanning continued initial therapy without chemotherapy; for non-responders, therapy was switched to 6 cycles of TCHP.

After 8 treatment cycles, 38% of group B responders achieved pathologic complete response (pCR). At a median follow-up of 43 months, the invasive disease-free survival (iDFS) was 94.8% in group B patients who underwent surgery (n=267), meeting the statistical requirement for significance. No new adverse reactions were seen.

- **U.S. Preventive Services Task Force (USPSTF) new guidelines for breast cancer screening**[27-29]

*The Task Force now recommends biennial screening for average-risk women who are aged 40 to 74.*

In 2016, the USPSTF recommended biennial mammograms for middle-aged women (age range, 50–74) with individualized decision-making for those who were aged 40 to 49.

The USPSTF now recommends

1. Biennial screening mammograms for women who are 40 to 74 and concluded with moderate certainty that such screening has a net benefit in preventing breast cancer–related mortality. An analysis estimated that this change will avert 1.3 additional breast cancer–related deaths per 1000 women screened biennially during a lifetime of screening — at the expense of an approximately 60% increase in false-positive results.
2. In women who are 75 or older, evidence was insufficient to recommend for or against screening.
3. For women with dense breasts, the Task Force found inadequate evidence to make a recommendation on benefits and harms of supplemental screening with ultrasound or magnetic resonance imaging after negative mammography.

- **Tumor-Infiltrating Lymphocytes (TILs) as a Prognostic Factor in Triple-Negative Breast Cancer**[31]

*Higher levels of TILs were associated with greater survival in patients who did not receive chemotherapy.*

Researchers conducted an international, retrospective, pooled analysis of individual patient-level data for almost 2000 patients (median age 56) with early-stage, triple-negative breast cancer (TNBC).

Among these patients, 60% had T1 lesions, 87% had node-negative disease, and 55% had stage 1 disease (T1cN0 tumors, 65%). No patients received systemic therapy; 61% underwent breast-conserving surgery and radiation therapy. TIL percentages were assessed in stromal tissue. The median TIL level was 15%; 34% of patients had TIL levels of at least 30%, and 21% had TIL levels of at least 50%. Higher TIL levels were associated with younger age and higher tumor grade. Median follow-up was 18 years.

Analyses were adjusted for age, tumor size and grade, nodal status, and receipt of radiation therapy. *Each* 10% higher TIL increment was associated with an 8% improvement in disease-free survival at 5 years, 10% improvement in relapse-free survival (RFS), 13% improvement in distant RFS, and 12% improvement in overall survival (OS).

- **Sentinel Node Biopsy Without Axillary Dissection in Patients with Sentinel-Node Metastases[32]**

*Survival was similar with and without complete axillary lymph node dissection in patients with clinically node-negative breast cancer and sentinel node metastases.*

In a randomized, phase 3, noninferiority trial (SENOMAC), researchers evaluated whether or not omitting axillary lymph node dissection (ALND) after a sentinel lymph node biopsy (SLNB) positive for breast cancer would worsen overall survival (OS). Patients with T1–3 tumors and one or two sentinel node macrometastases (>2 mm) were eligible, as were those who had additional micrometastases or who had extracapsular nodal extension.

Of the 2540 patients in the trial, 40% were aged 65 or older, 94% had T1 or T2 tumors, 64% had breast-conserving surgery, 70% had one or two sentinel nodes removed, and 87% had luminal ER+/HER2− tumors. Approximately one third of patients had extracapsular nodal extension. Approximately 65% of patients received adjuvant chemotherapy, 88% received postoperative regional nodal radiation therapy, 93% received adjuvant endocrine therapy, and 9% received HER2-directed therapy. The median follow-up was 46.8 months.

The estimated 5-year OS, the primary endpoint, was similar in the ALND- and SLNB-only arms (92% and 93%). The two arms also had similar 5-year breast cancer–specific survival (97%) and 5-year recurrence-free survival (89% and 90%).

These results indicated that patients undergoing SLNB alone have outcomes similar to those also undergoing complete ALND.

- **A New Adjuvant Regimen for Patients with Early Breast Cancer: Interim Results**[36]

*Adding ribociclib to endocrine therapy improved disease–free survival in a diverse group of patients with estrogen-receptor (ER) positive, HER2−negative early breast cancer.*

Researchers reported prespecified interim results with ribociclib in an open-label, randomized, phase 3 trial involving 5101 patients with ER+/HER2− early breast cancer (EBC) which was defined as anatomical stage II/III disease. Ribocciclib is a cyclin dependent kinase inhibitor.

Treatments were

1. A nonsteroidal aromatase inhibitor (NSAI; anastrozole or letrozole) alone for 5 years

or

2. A nonsteroidal aromatase inhibitor with ribociclib (dosage, 400 mg daily; 21 days on and 7 days off) for 3 years. The GnRH analog goserelin was required for gonadal suppression in men and premenopausal women. Patients with stage IIB/III disease were eligible irrespective of nodal status; those with stage IIa had at least one involved node, a grade 3 tumor, or grade 2 disease with high proliferation or high genomic risk.

More than 99% of participants were women (>50% postmenopausal). At a median follow-up of 34 months, 78% of combination recipients were still receiving at least one treatment. At 3 years, disease-free survival (DFS) was 90.4% in the ribociclib plus NSAI group and 87.1% in the NSAI-alone group, a statistically significant lower risk for an event with the addition of ribociclib. Numerically, distant DFS and overall survival also favored adding ribociclib.

- **Targeting the Androgen Receptor in Breast Cancer[41]**

*The selective androgen receptor (AR) modulator enobosarm showed activity in a small study of patients with ER-positive/AR-positive metastatic breast cancer.*

Recent studies have shown that the androgen receptor (AR) is a tumor suppressor and AR agonists can lead to AR activation and antitumor activity in estrogen receptor (ER)–positive breast cancer. Selective AR modulators (SARMs) selectively bind to the AR without causing the virilizing effects associated with androgen therapy and AR antagonists. Enobosarm is an oral SARM that has demonstrated in vivo antitumor activity in ER-positive and ER-resistant breast cancer.

In a multinational, randomized, open-label, phase 2 trial researchers assessed the effects of enobosarm at two dose levels (9 mg or 18 mg daily) in 136 postmenopausal patients with ER-positive/AR-positive metastatic breast cancer. The median age was 60.5 years and 62.5 years in the 9 mg and 18 mg groups, respectively. Overall, 92% of patients had received prior chemotherapy and 82% had received endocrine therapy (median, two lines) in the metastatic disease setting. Median follow-up was 7.5 months.

The clinical benefit rate at 24 weeks was 32% in the 9-mg group and 29% in the 18-mg group. Most treatment-related toxicity was grade 1 or 2. Grade 3 or 4 treatment-related toxicity occurred in 8% of the 9-mg group and 16% of the 18-mg group, most commonly elevated hepatic transaminases, hypercalcemia, and fatigue.

This study shows that enobosarm has antitumor activity in patients with heavily pretreated, ER-positive, metastatic breast cancer and is well tolerated. Further studies are required to determine the optimal dosage and the optimal duration of treatment.

- **Are Taxanes Safe for Pregnant Patients with Breast Cancer?[53,54]**

*A retrospective study suggested that administration of taxanes after the first trimester is safe for mothers and infants.*

In a retrospective, international study, researchers assessed maternal and neonatal adverse events associated with use of taxanes during pregnancy in patients with breast cancer. Of 103 patients, 77% had stage II or III disease. Paclitaxel was the most commonly administered taxane (96%), mostly at a dose of 80 $mg/m^2$ weekly. The median gestational age at initiation of taxane therapy was 28 weeks.

The prevalence of maternal adverse events was low (grade 3 - 4, 6.8%) and similar to that expected in a nonpregnant breast cancer population. Despite the need to administer steroids with paclitaxel, the prevalence of gestational diabetes (5.3%) and hypertensive disorders of pregnancy (4.3%) was not increased relative to the general population.

The live birth rate was 98% with a median gestational age of 37 weeks. Overall, 43% of infants were born preterm (<37 weeks), which is higher than in the general population but comparable to the rate reported with use of anthracycline-based chemotherapy in pregnancy. Importantly, the rate of congenital malformations was similar to that in the general population (~2%). Among 28 infants followed for a median of 42 months, 24 were reported as healthy. This report offers reassurance regarding the safety of paclitaxel administered beyond the first trimester. For appropriate pregnant patients at significant risk for breast cancer recurrence based on clinical features, a sequential anthracycline-taxane regimen could be considered.

- **Risk for Invasive Breast Cancer and Mortality After Ductal Carcinoma In Situ (DCIS)[55,56]**

*This study suggested that more frequent surveillance may result in better outcomes for patients with DCIS.*

Investigators evaluated the risk for invasive cancer in >27,000 women in England diagnosed with DCIS outside the NHS screening program from 1990 to 2018. Of these, 3,651 women were eventually diagnosed with invasive breast cancer; the incidence rate of 13.28/1000 woman-years was 4 times greater than expected from incidence rates in the general population. The risk was elevated, and similar, across all age groups and throughout follow-up. The 25-year cumulative risk of breast cancer death ranged from 5.8% in those aged 45–49 years at diagnosis to 7.6% in those aged <45 years. Overall, the risk of death was 4 times higher than in the general population.

**Mammography Preferences Among Women in Their 40s[73]**

*A survey suggested that many women might prefer to delay screening for breast cancer*

Researchers conducted a survey in 2022 to assess attitudes toward screening among a diverse group of 495 average-risk U.S. women (aged 39–49). Preference to initiate or delay mammography was determined before and after patients viewed a decision aid with information on mammography benefits and harms and completed a personal risk assessment.

Most participants indicated a preference to proceed with screening; however, 27% preferred to delay (either until older but before age 50 or until age 50) even before viewing the decision aid. This proportion increased significantly to 38% after viewing the decision aid. Participants who preferred to delay screening had a lower breast cancer risk overall.

- **Overall Survival with Pembrolizumab in Early-Stage Triple-Negative Breast Cancer[83]**

*In patients with early-stage triple-negative (ER-, PR-, Her-2-) breast cancer, a trial showed significant improvements in pathological complete response and event-free survival with the addition of pembrolizumab to chemotherapy*

Patients with previously untreated stage II or III triple-negative breast cancer were randomized to receive neoadjuvant therapy with four cycles of pembrolizumab (at a dose of 200 mg) or placebo every 3 weeks plus paclitaxel and carboplatin, followed by four cycles of pembrolizumab or placebo plus doxorubicin–cyclophosphamide or epirubicin–cyclophosphamide. After definitive surgery, patients received adjuvant pembrolizumab (pembrolizumab–chemotherapy group) or placebo (placebo–chemotherapy group) every 3 weeks for up to nine cycles.

The estimated overall survival at 60 months was 86.6% in the pembrolizumab–chemotherapy group, compared with 81.7% in the placebo–chemotherapy group (p=0.002).

- **Trastuzumab Deruxtecan after Endocrine Therapy in Metastatic Breast Cancer[84]**

*In patients with hormone receptor–positive, HER2-low or HER2-ultralow metastatic breast cancer who had received one or more lines of endocrine-based therapy, treatment with trastuzumab deruxtecan resulted in longer progression-free survival than chemotherapy.*

In patients with HER2-low disease, the median progression-free survival was 13.2 months in the trastuzumab deruxtecan group and 8.1 months in the chemotherapy group (p<0.001).

- **Predicting Benefit from Ovarian Suppression in Young Women with High-Risk Breast Cancer[93]**

*In this study the results suggested that suppression of ovarian function will be of benefit in young, high-risk patients with breast cancer index (BCI) (H/I)-low tumors, but not in those with BCI(H/I)-high tumors.*

Genomic assays are used to determine which patients with early stage, estrogen-receptor–positive (ER+) breast cancer can avoid chemotherapy and to indicate the optimal duration of adjuvant endocrine therapy. One such tool, the Breast Cancer Index (BCI), is composed of two biomarker panels: the *HOXB13/IL17BR* (H/I) gene ratio, which is a measure of estrogen signalling, and the 5-gene Molecular Grade Index, which is a measure of tumor proliferation. Clinical trials have shown that patients with BCI (H/I)-high tumors benefit significantly from extended duration of endocrine therapy after 5 years, while those with BCI (H/I)-low tumors do not.

The previously reported Suppression of Ovarian Function Trial (SOFT) demonstrated that compared to tamoxifen alone, exemestane or tamoxifen in combination with ovarian function suppression (OFS) improved both disease-free survival (DFS) and overall survival at 12 years in premenopausal women. (Ovarian function suppression can be achieved with the gonadotropin-releasing–hormone agonist triptorelin, bilateral oophorectomy, or bilateral ovarian radiation).

In the current study, researchers performed the BCI test using RNA extracted from tumor samples available for 1687 of the 3047 SOFT participants. Of these patients, 53% remained premenopausal after chemotherapy, and 66% were node negative.

The investigators postulated that patients with BCI (H/I)-high tumors would be most likely to benefit from OFS. However, patients with BCI (H/I)-high tumors (n=715) gained no benefit from OFS, while those with BCI(H/I)-low tumors (n=972) had significant benefit. The 12-year absolute benefit in breast cancer–free interval with OFS plus tamoxifen or exemestane versus tamoxifen alone was as follows:

1. BCI (H/I)-high: tamoxifen/OFS, −1.2%; exemestane/OFS, −0.4%
2. BCI (H/I)-low: tamoxifen/OFS, 7.3%; exemestane/OFS, 11.6%

- **Supplemental MRI for Women with Dense Breasts[94]**

*Supplemental MRI appears to avert a small number of deaths but would increase false-positive recalls substantially, and harm–benefit trade-offs appear to be most favorable with biennial screening starting at age 50.*

Digital breast tomosynthesis (DBT) is emerging as the standard of care for breast imaging based on improvements in both screening and diagnostic imaging outcomes. The quasi three-dimensional information obtained from the reconstructed DBT data set allows a more efficient imaging work-up than imaging with two-dimensional full-field digital mammography alone.

In this study researchers used well-established models to simulate outcomes if magnetic resonance imaging (MRI) were added to digital breast tomosynthesis (DBT) based on breast density. They projected the following:

1. Biennial DBT screening for middle-aged women (age range 50–74) would result in 7.4 breast cancer deaths averted and 884 false-positive recalls per 1000 women during lifetime screening. Adding biennial MRI for women with *extremely dense* breasts would increase deaths averted by 0.1 and false-positive recalls by 35. Extending MRI to women with *heterogeneously dense* breasts would lead to an additional 0.5 deaths averted and 170 additional false-positive recalls.
2. Starting the above-stated scenarios at age 40 rather than age 50 would lead to similar increases in deaths averted but larger increases in false-positive recalls.
3. Annual screening would increase the number of deaths averted slightly but would more than double rates of false positives.

## CHAPTER 2. LUNG CANCER

### 2.1. NON-SMALL CELL LUNG CANCER (NSCLC)

- **First-line combination therapy for EGFR-mutated NSCLC[1]**

*Amivantamab plus lazertinib increased progression-free survival compared with osimertinib alone in patients with previously untreated, locally advanced or metastatic EGFR-mutated NSCLC.*

Mutations of the epithelial growth factor receptor (EGFR) occur in 15% of NSCLC cases and have a significant effect on their response to treatment since NSCLCs with such a mutation are responsive to tyrosine kinase inhibitors (TKIs). Osimertib and lazertrinib are TKIs, while amibantimab is a EGFR/MET bispecific monoclonal antibody. MET is a tyrosine kinase receptor for hepatocyte growth factor. In this study, investigators found that amivantamab plus lazertinib increased progression-free survival compared with osimertinib alone in patients with previously untreated, locally advanced or metastatic EGFR-mutated NSCLC.

However, it is likely that many patients and clinicians will opt for osimertinib alone as initial treatment, given the increased time, costs, and toxicities associated with more-intensive combination therapy. Further trials are thus needed to determine the optimal dosages and the optimal duration of treatment of the combination of amivantamab plus lazertinib versus osimertinib.

- **Targeted therapy after chemoradiation for unresectable stage III NSCLC[2]**

*A new standard of care for unresectable stage III NSCLC.*

Researchers reported that progression-free survival (PFS), the primary endpoint, was significantly improved with osimertinib compared with placebo (median, 39.1 vs. 5.6 months; hazard ratio, 0.16; $p<0.001$). Two hundred and sixteen adult patients with locally advanced, unresectable stage III NSCLC with an epithelial growth factor receptor (EGFR) exon 19 deletion or L858R mutation, who did not experience progression following definitive chemoradiotherapy, were randomized to either the osimertinib or placebo. Treatment with osimertinib improved progression-free survival compared to placebo in patients with unresectable stage III NSCLC harboring an EGFR mutation. Progression-free survival (PFS), the primary endpoint, was significantly improved with osimertinib compared with placebo (median, 39.1 vs. 5.6 months; hazard ratio, 0.16; $P<0.001$). This result was considered to be a new standard of care for unresectable stage III NSCLC.

- **Perioperative Nivolumab Improves Survival in Resectable NSCLC**[19]

*Event-free survival was longer with the addition of perioperative nivolumab to neoadjuvant chemotherapy than with the addition of placebo in patients with stage II and III disease.*

While it has been shown that neoadjuvant chemoimmunotherapy improves survival compared with chemotherapy alone in non–small-cell lung cancer (NSCLC), whether postoperative immunotherapy would further improve outcomes was explored. In this phase 3 trial, 461 patients with resectable stage II and III NSCLC without known *EGFR* mutations or *ALK* translocations were randomized to receive neoadjuvant chemotherapy plus either nivolumab or placebo (every 3 weeks for 4 cycles), followed by surgery, followed by adjuvant nivolumab or placebo (every 4 weeks for 1 year).

Event-free survival (the primary outcome) at 18 months was significantly higher in the nivolumab group than the placebo group (70.2% vs. 50.0%; hazard ratio, 0.58; $p<0.001$); median event-free survival was not reached versus 18.4 months, respectively. Pathological complete response occurred in 25.3% of patients in the nivolumab group compared with 4.7% in the placebo group.

In subgroup analyses, event-free survival was improved with postoperative nivolumab across categories of tumor PD-L1 expression, with greater magnitude of benefit in patients with higher PD-L1 expression.

Of note, chemotherapy was cisplatin-based in 24% versus 18% of patients in the nivolumab and placebo groups, respectively, and was carboplatin-based in 73% versus 78%. Grade 3 or 4 treatment-related adverse events occurred in 32.5%

versus 25.2% of the nivolumab and placebo groups. Treatment-related adverse events led to treatment discontinuation in 19.3% versus 7.4% of patients, respectively.

- **Adjuvant Alectinib vs. Chemotherapy in *ALK*-Positive Non–Small-Cell Lung Cancer[30]**

*Alectinib improved disease-free survival compared with chemotherapy in patients with early stage, resected ALK-positive NSCLC.*

Mutations in the anaplastic lymphoma kinase (*ALK*) gene occur in about 5% of patients with non–small-cell lung cancer (NSCLC). These patients are more likely than those with other types of NSCLC to be aged ≤55 years, to be never smokers, and to develop central nervous system (CNS) metastases. Alectinib, a kinase inhibitor, is currently approved for the first-line treatment of advanced *ALK*-positive NSCLC.

This international, open-label, phase 3 trial (ALINA) assessed the efficacy and safety of 24 months of adjuvant alectinib versus platinum-based chemotherapy in 257 patients with completely resected stage IB to IIIA *ALK*-positive NSCLC. The primary endpoint was disease-free survival (DFS). Patients were randomized to receive oral alectinib (600 mg twice daily) for 24 months or chemotherapy (cisplatin and vinorelbine, gemcitabine, or pemetrexed) for four 21-day cycles.

Treatment with alectinib reduced the risk of recurrence or death by 76% (hazard ratio, 0.24; 95% CI, 0.13–0.45; $p<0.001$) compared with adjuvant chemotherapy alone. The alectinib group also had a 78% improvement in central nervous system DFS (HR, 0.22; 95% CI, 0.08–0.58).

Alectinib was well tolerated with no new safety signals. Adverse events led to alectinib dose reduction in 25.8% of patients and to early discontinuation of adjuvant alectinib therapy in 5.5%.

The substantial improvement in DFS makes adjuvant alectinib a new standard of care for patients with resected *ALK*-positive NSCLC and underscores the need for molecular testing in NSCLC, regardless of stage.

- **Lung Cancer Screening Complications**[64]

*Low-dose computed tomography screening has higher rates of subsequent procedures than previously reported.*

In the National Lung Screening Trial, low-dose computed tomography (LDCT) lowered lung cancer–specific mortality among smokers although the number of people needed to screen was 320 to order to prevent 1 death. Additionally, many screened patients required additional imaging or procedures, and some developed procedural complications. I

In this study, investigators retrospectively assessed more than 9,000 patients from five large U.S. healthcare systems who received LDCT screening in routine clinical practice. Sixteen percent of LDCTs showed abnormalities, and 1.5% of patients were diagnosed with lung cancer within 12 months.

Study findings included the following:

1. LDCT's sensitivity was 93%, specificity was 84%, positive predictive value was 10%, and negative predictive value was 99.8%.
2. Among screened patients, one third underwent further imaging (i.e., additional CT, magnetic resonance imaging, or positron-emission tomography), and 1 in 35 patients underwent invasive procedures (i.e., biopsy, bronchoscopy, mediastinoscopy, thoracoscopy, thoracentesis, or thoracotomy).

Compared with complication rates in the National Lung Screening Trial, this study had approximately twice the rate of procedural complications (31% vs. 18%) and major complications (i.e., acute respiratory failure, lung collapse or cardiac arrest; 21% vs. 9%).

This study's results might complicate discussions with patients regarding potential screening risks. Nevertheless, the high rate of long-term, cancer-free survival among patients with cancer detected by screening currently supports guideline-recommended screening that includes shared decision-making.

- **An Effective New Tyrosine Kinase Inhibitor for *ROS1* Fusion-Positive Non–Small-Cell Lung Cancer**[67]

*Repotrectinib is a new standard of care for these patients.*

*ROS1* fusions occur in 2% of non–small-cell lung cancers (NSCLCs) and represent a targetable oncogene. Although two highly active ROS1 tyrosine kinase inhibitors (TKIs), crizotinib and entrectinib, have been available for some years, resistance inevitably develops — often via on-target *ROS1* mutations such as G2032R. Additionally, they have limited central nervous system efficacy. Thus, this there is a need for more effective therapies. Repotrectinib is a next-generation ROS1 and NTRK TKI that was designed to inhibit both wild type and G2032R-mutant *ROS1* and to have significant central nervous system (CNS) efficacy.

In this international phase 1–2 trial, investigators assessed the efficacy and safety of repotrectinib in patients with *ROS1* fusion-positive NSCLC. The primary efficacy population included 71 patients who had not previously received a ROS1 TKI and 56 patients who had received a ROS1 TKI and had never received chemotherapy.

An objective response occurred in 79% of the TKI-naive patients; median progression free-survival was 35.7 months. In the patients previously treated with a ROS1 TKI, 38% had an objective response and median progression-free survival was 9.0 months. Notably, 59% of the 17 patients with acquired *ROS1* G2032R mutations demonstrated a response. Intracranial responses were noted across all cohorts.

The safety analysis included 426 patients who were treated with the phase 2 dose. The most common treatment-related adverse events of any grade were dizziness (58%), dysgeusia (50%), and paresthesia (30%), which were managed by supportive care, dose reduction, or both. The most common clinically significant grade 3 or higher adverse events were anemia (4%) and dizziness (3%).

- **Improving Equity in Lung Cancer Screening Eligibility**[109]

*Using duration of smoking, rather than pack-years, might eliminate the current racial disparity.*

In a retrospective U.S. study, researchers analyzed two large cohorts with data on smoking history and incidence of lung cancer. The hypothetical performance of the standard ≥20-pack-year screening criterion was compared with a proposed ≥20-year smoking-duration criterion.

Among patients in one cohort who eventually developed lung cancer, 58% of Black patients and 74% of white patients would have qualified for screening under the pack-year criterion. These proportions increased to 85% and 82%, respectively, under the smoking-duration criterion, which is a substantial improvement in sensitivity and eliminates the racial disparity. In the second cohort (comprised exclusively of Black patients), a smoking-duration criterion would have been more sensitive for predicting eventual lung cancer.

## 2.2. SMALL CELL LUNG CANCER

### Durvalumab after Chemoradiotherapy in Limited-Stage Small-Cell Lung Cancer[81]

*Adjuvant therapy with durvalumab led to significantly longer overall survival and progression-free survival than placebo among patients with limited-stage small-cell lung cancer.*

In a phase 3, double-blind, randomized, placebo-controlled trial, investigators assigned patients with limited stage small cell lung cancer who did not have progression after standard cisplatin chemotherapy to receive durvalumab at a dose of 1500 mg, durvalumab (1500 mg) plus tremelimumab at a dose of 75 mg (four doses only), or placebo every 4 weeks for up to 24 months. Randomization was stratified according to disease stage (I or II vs. III) and receipt of prophylactic cranial irradiation (yes vs. no). (Durvalumab and tremelimumab are both immune checkpoint inhibitors, although they block different molecules: durvalumab inhibits PDL-1, while tremelimumab blocks CTLA-4).

Results of the first planned interim analysis of the two primary end points of overall survival and progression-free survival with durvalumab as compared with placebo showed that durvalumab therapy led to significantly longer overall survival than placebo (median, 55.9 months vs. 33.4 months) (p=0.01), as well as to significantly longer progression-free survival (median 16.6 months vs. 9.2 months (p=0.02).

The outcomes in the durvalumab–tremelimumab group remain blinded.

## Chapter 3. COLORECTAL CANCER[10]

- *Results from a study indicate near-universal response to immune checkpoint inhibitors in patients with locally advanced microsatellite instability–high (MSI-high) colorectal cancers.*

Investigators reported the results of the NICHE-2 trial, a phase 2 trial treating 115 patients with MSI-high colon cancer which was clinical stage II or III.

Patients received one dose of ipilimumab (1 mg/kg) and two doses of nivolumab (3 mg/kg; days 1 and 15), followed by surgical resection. Thirty-seven patients had hereditary Lynch syndrome. The cancer was clinical stage T3/4a in 21%, stage T4a/T4b in 65%, and clinical node–positive in 67%.

The primary safety endpoint of reaching timely surgery was achieved in 98% of patients; surgery was delayed in only two patients, due to therapy toxicity. At a median follow-up of 26.2 months, 98% of 111 eligible patients achieved a pathologic response (i.e., <50% of viable tumor cells found), 95% had a major pathologic response (<10% of viable tumor cells), and 68% had a pathologic complete response. Adjuvant chemotherapy was considered in 14 patients with residual nodal disease found at surgery but was administered to only three. Five patients had grade 3 or 4 adverse events related to immunotherapy. No recurrences were observed.

- **Chemotherapy regimen before liver surgery predicts development of steatohepatitis and risk for 90-day mortality[13]**

*Chemotherapy before resection of liver metastatic disease – oxaliplatin versus irinotecan*

With effective oxaliplatin- or irinotecan-based regimens, approximately 13% of patients with initially unresectable disease can be treated successfully with liver surgery because of substantial downsizing of hepatic colorectal metastases.

In a cohort of 406 patients, 248 of whom received preoperative chemotherapy, investigators demonstrated that different drugs cause different types of liver injury. Irinotecan, compared with no chemotherapy, was associated with increased risk of steatohepatitis (20.2% vs. 4.4%; $p<0.001$); oxaliplatin, compared with no chemotherapy, was associated with increased risk for sinusoidal dilatation (18.9% vs. 1.9%; $p<0.001$).

The most important finding was that development of steatohepatitis was associated with worse postoperative outcomes. Steatohepatitis was the sole liver injury associated with increased risk for death by 90 days after hepatectomy (14.7% vs. 1.6% in patients without steatohepatitis ($p=0.001$). The risk of steatohepatitis after irinotecan treatment was higher in patients with body-mass indices of ≥25 $kg/m^2$ compared to those with lower BMIs.

- **In patients receiving FOLFIRI/cetuximab, maintenance cetuximab was not noninferior to continued combination treatment[14]**

  *Cetuximab maintenance showed a nonsignificant trend toward superiority in overall survival compared to cetuximab combined with cytotoxic chemotherapy.*

Investigators reported results of an open-label, phase 3 maintenance trial for patients with *RAS/BRAF* wild-type metastatic CRC who were randomized to either FOLFIRI/cetuximab until disease progression or FOLFIRI/cetuximab for 4 months followed by maintenance with cetuximab alone (ERMES trial). Of 593 patients treated, 337 patients with response or stable disease at 4 months (57%) proceeded to therapy continuation or maintenance cetuximab. Most patients had undergone surgery (61%), had one metastatic disease site (80%), and had left-sided (71%) versus right-sided (19%) primary tumors.

The primary endpoint of noninferior PFS was not met for cetuximab compared with FOLFIRI/cetuximab (median, 10.0 vs. 12.2 months; hazard ratio, 1.3), exceeding the study's noninferiority boundary. Grades 3 and 4 adverse events during the maintenance phase were numerically more common with FOLFIRI/cetuximab (35.1%) than with cetuximab alone (20.2%). Rates of overall response were similar for the two arms (67.5% and 71.6%, respectively). Cetuximab maintenance showed a nonsignificant trend toward superiority in overall survival (cetuximab 35.7 months; FOLFIRI/cetuximab, 30.7 months; HR, 0.79; *p*=0.119).

- **Neoadjuvant Chemotherapy in Colon Cancer Is Safe and Feasible[24]**

*Preoperative chemotherapy was associated with modest pathologic downsizing and better overall survival than postoperative-only chemotherapy in a phase III trial.*

In the OPTICAL trial, investigators in China randomized patients to 3 months of preoperative chemotherapy (with either mFOLFOX6 [fluorouracil, leucovorin, oxaliplatin] or CAPOX [capecitabine and oxaliplatin]) followed by 3 months of postoperative chemotherapy or to 6 months of chemotherapy all administered postoperatively. Of the 744 evaluable patients, 25% had clinical stage T3 cancer on CT scan, 75% had stage T4, 77% had node-positive status, and 56% had left-sided primary cancers. In the preoperative group, 70% received mFOLFOX6, and 30% received CAPOX; overall, 58% completed preoperative therapy. Adjuvant therapy was started after surgery in 83% of the preoperative group and 80% of the postoperative-only group.

At a median follow-up of 48 months, 3-year disease-free survival, the primary endpoint, was not significantly improved in the preoperative group compared with the postoperative-only group (82.1% vs. 77.5%; hazard ratio, 0.74; *p*=0.07). However, subgroup analyses suggested a more pronounced benefit of preoperative therapy among female patients (86.5% vs. 75.3%; HR, 0.54). Among all patients, the preoperative group had significantly better 3-year overall survival than the postoperative-only group (95.1% vs. 89.6%; HR 0.44; *p*=0.01) and modest pathologic downstaging, with 7% of patients achieving a pathologic complete response. Rates of grade 3/4 serious adverse events were similar in both groups.

This trial demonstrated that administering 3 months of preoperative chemotherapy in clinically staged colon cancer is safe and feasible.

- **Primary Tumor Resection Does Not Improve Survival in Metastatic Colon Cancer[33]**

*Results from the pooled analysis of two European trials support the avoidance of primary tumor resection in patients presenting with metastatic colon cancer and inoperable metastases. The high rate of failure to administer any palliative chemotherapy in the upfront surgery group underscores that primary surgery should continue to be reserved for patients with bleeding or obstructing tumors.*

Initial surgery for patients with metastatic colon cancer is warranted when the primary tumor is bleeding or obstructing. However, for patients with asymptomatic tumors and metastases not amenable to curative resection, results from retrospective, phase 2 and phase 3 trials have varied, with some supporting and others questioning a survival benefit for upfront surgery. Investigators now report combined results from the SYNCHRONOUS and CCRe-IV randomized trials comparing upfront primary tumor resection (PTR) followed by chemotherapy to treatment with chemotherapy alone in patients with colon cancer and metastatic disease not curable with surgery.

Of the 393 patients, 95% had liver metastases. Primary tumors were left-sided in 53% of patients and right-sided in 45%. 45% received an oxaliplatin-fluoropyrimidine doublet chemotherapy, 35% the addition of bevacizumab, and 18% an EGFR-targeting antibody. The median follow-up was 36.7 months. The primary endpoint of median overall survival was similar in the two groups (PTR, 16.7 months; no-PTR, 18.6 months). Chemotherapy was not given to 24% of patients in the PTR group and 6% of the no-PTR group. The no-PTR group had a significantly higher rate of serious adverse events (18%) than the PTR group (10%), due to more ileus or bowel obstruction (no-PTR group, 18 patients; PTR group, 2 patients).

- **A Blood Test for Cancer DNA: An Eventual New Option for Colorectal Cancer Screening?**[43]

*This test detected 88% of early-stage colorectal cancers but sensitivity for advanced precancerous lesions was low.*

In this study researchers examined the performance of a cell-free DNA blood test (which is not yet approved as a screening test by the U.S. FDA) in 7,861 people who also were undergoing colonoscopy. The test yielded the following results:

1. It detected 88% of stage I, II, or III (not yet metastatic) colorectal cancers.
2. It detected 13% of advanced precancerous lesions.
3. It was falsely positive in 10% of people who did not have colorectal cancer or advanced precancerous lesions.

This cell-free DNA blood test was less accurate than the multitarget stool DNA test (which also includes an assay for fecal hemoglobin). However, the blood test only requires venipuncture and thus might attract some people who do not wish to have initial screening with colonoscopy or stool testing.

- **Positive Fecal Immunochemical Test and Negative Colonoscopy: Should Upper Endoscopy Be Next?**[95]

*When this scenario occurs during screening, the incidence of upper endoscopy–detectable cancer is very low, but not zero*

Investigators used data from a colo-rectal cancer screening registry that included about 2 million middle-aged or older patients (age range 55–75) who were screened with quantitative fecal immunochemical tests (FIT). The threshold for positivity of the FIT test is 47 µg hemoglobin/g of feces.

They found the following:

1. About 3% of patients were FIT-positive with negative colonoscopy, 3% were FIT-positive with advanced neoplasia (advanced adenoma or colorectal cancer), and 94% were FIT-negative.
2. The 3-year incidence of cancers proximal to the colon was slightly (but statistically significantly) higher in FIT-positive than in FIT-negative patients (≈0.6% vs. 0.4%).
3. The 3-year incidence of cancers potentially detectable by esophagogastroduodenoscopy (EGD) also was higher in FIT-positive patients than in FIT-negative patients (0.4% vs. 0.2%).
4. Among FIT-positive patients, the incidence of cancers proximal to the colon was similar in patients with or without advanced colorectal neoplasia.

- **Benefits from Adjuvant Treatment for Colon Cancer in Older vs. Younger Patients**[110]

*In patients aged 70 and older with stage III colon cancer, time to recurrence was similar to that in younger patients.*

Debate continues as to whether oxaliplatin should be added to adjuvant chemotherapy in older patients. In a combined analysis of 12 randomized trials in the IDEA and ACCENT trial databases, investigators compared outcomes between patients aged ≥70 and <70 years.

Of nearly 18,000 patients, 24% were ≥70 years; compared to younger patients, they were more frequently male and had ECOG PS >1, T4 tumors located in the proximal colon, microsatellite-instability–high status, and BRAFV600E mutations. More patients <70 than >70 received 6 months of fluorouracil, leucovorin, and oxaliplatin (FOLFOX; 51.9% vs. 39.4%), whereas more patients >70 received capecitabine and oxaliplatin (CAPOX) either for 3 months (17.5% vs. 13.2%) or 6 months (22.0% vs.18.5%).

At a median follow-up of 75.8 months, multivariate analysis showed no significant difference in time to recurrence between age groups overall or between age groups among those treated with 6-month or 3-month regimens. However, disease-free survival (DFS) and overall survival (OS) were shorter in the older group overall and among the 6-month and 3-month groups. Among older patients, time to recurrence was shorter with 3 versus 6 months of treatment (hazard ratio, 1.19; p=0.012), but therapy duration had no effect on DFS or OS.

Rates of early treatment discontinuation were higher in patients >70 than in those <70 (22.0% vs. 15.5%; p<0.001), especially among patients who received 6-month regimens (28.9% vs. 19.0%; p< 0.001). Among patients treated with CAPOX, those >70 had higher rates of diarrhea, neutropenia, and mucositis.

## CHAPTER 4. ANAL CANCER

- **Atezolizumab Added to Chemotherapy Fails to Improve Outcomes in Anal Cancer[23]**

*The addition of atezolizumab (an immune checkpoint inhibitor) to modified docetaxel, cisplatin, and fluorouracil chemotherapy did not improve survival or response rates compared with chemotherapy alone.*

Investigators in France reported results of an open-label, phase 2 trial evaluating the addition of atezolizumab to first-line chemotherapy with a modified schedule of docetaxel, cisplatin and 5-fluorouracil (mDCF). Patients with metastatic anal cancer were randomized to receive mDCF (docetaxel 40 mg/m$^2$ and cisplatin 40 mg/m$^2$ for 1 day and 5-FU 1200 mg/m$^2$ per day for 2 days every 2 weeks) either alone or combined with atezolizumab (800 mg cycled every 2 weeks). Of the 97 patients, 73% were female; 41% had synchronous (occurring at the same time) metastases and 37% had metachronous (occurring at different times) metastases; 51% had received prior chemoradiotherapy; and nearly half had liver and distant lymph node metastases.

The primary endpoint of progression-free survival (PFS) at 12 months was not improved with the addition of atezolizumab compared with chemotherapy alone (45% vs. 43%). There was also no difference in median PFS (9.4 vs. 8.7 months, respectively), 12-month overall survival (77% vs. 81%), or response rate (75% vs. 78%). In the subset of patients with combined positive PD-L1 scores (CPS) ≥5%, 12-month PFS was higher with atezolizumab than with chemotherapy alone. Rates of grade 3/4 serious adverse events were higher with atezolizumab compared with chemotherapy alone (61% vs. 42%).

The addition of the immune checkpoint inhibitor atezolizumab to first-line chemotherapy in patients with metastatic anal cancer did not improve outcomes over chemotherapy alone. The observation of a potential benefit for atezolizumab in patients with CPS ≥5% is hypothesis-generating and requires confirmation in other trials.

## CHAPTER 5. PROSTATE CANCER

- **Long-Term Outcomes with Structured Active Surveillance of Low-Grade Prostate Cancer[15]**

*During 7 years of follow-up, approximately half the patients in this study maintained their low-grade classification, and only 0.1% died of prostate cancer.*

In a prospective observational study, researchers at 10 U.S. and Canadian academic medical centers enrolled 2,155 men (median age, 63) who were managed with active surveillance. About 85% of the cases were classified as low or very low risk, and 15% were classified as favorable intermediate risk. Protocol-directed follow-up involved prostate-specific antigen (PSA) testing every 3 to 6 months, confirmatory biopsies at 6 to 12 months after diagnosis, and subsequent biopsies every 2 years after diagnosis. Adherence to the protocol was roughly 90%.

At a median follow-up of 7.2 years, about half of patients maintained their low-grade classification and received no treatment. Cancer grade was reclassified in 43% of participants, and 49% underwent radiotherapy or surgery. Progression to metastatic cancer occurred in 21 patients (1%), and 3 patients died of prostate cancer.

Although a fairly high proportion of these patients were eventually reclassified to having higher-grade disease, an important finding is that about half were *not* reclassified, and only 0.1% died of metastatic disease.

- **Androgen-Deprivation Therapy (ADT) Use and Duration in Postoperative Patients with Prostate Cancer[16]**

*Clinicians and patients need to consider the risks for ADT-related toxicities in decision making.*

Radiotherapy (RT) combined with androgen-deprivation therapy (ADT) has long been the established standard of care for treating patients with localized or locally advanced prostate cancer. However, in men with biochemical failure after prostatectomy, the role of this combination is less well established. To learn more, investigators conducted RADICALS-HD, an international, multicenter study of post-prostatectomy patients with PSA values less than 5 ng/mL and no metastatic disease on bone scan or computed tomography.

Although the study was designed as a three-way randomization of patients receiving RT, the researchers later chose to separately evaluate two comparisons: RT alone versus RT plus short-course ADT (SC-ADT; 6 months), and RT plus SC-ADT versus RT plus long-course ADT (LC; 24 months). Each study randomized approximately 1500 patients, with a median age of about 66, median PSA values of 0.21 to 0.23, and median follow-up of 9 years.

In the first comparison, 10 year metastasis-free survival (MFS) was 79% in the RT-only group and 80% in the RT+SC-ADT group. Toxicity of grade 3 or higher was observed in 17% of the RT-only group and 14% of the RT+SC-ADT group.

In the second comparison, 10-year MFS was 72% in the RT+SC-ADT group and 78% in the RT+LC-ADT group, which was a statistically significant difference. Toxicity of grade 3 or higher was observed in 14% of the RT+SC-ADT group and 19% of the RT+LC-ADT group.

No treatment-related deaths occurred.

These reports from RADICALS-HD add important data to help clinicians make therapy recommendations for patients with post-prostatectomy biochemical failure. Although MFS findings slightly favored LC-ADT over SC-ADT, clinicians and patients need to consider the risks for ADT-related toxicities in decision making.

- **Prostate Cancer Screening Guidelines for Black Men[25]**

*The Prostate Cancer Foundation has issued the first set of stand-alone guidelines for prostate cancer screening screening for Black men in the U.S.A.*

Black men have both an extremely high incidence of prostate cancer and a significantly higher lifetime risk of dying from it compared with other groups. Current screening guidelines typically include recommendations regarding Black men, but the recommendations are somewhat variable.

A multidisciplinary panel conducted a comprehensive evidence-based systematic review and selected 264 studies deemed relevant for addressing 6 key questions regarding screening of Black men in the U.S.A. for prostate cancer screening.

Key recommendations were

1. Black men should be screened for prostate cancer as the benefits generally outweigh the risks.
2. Prostate-specific antigen (PSA) testing is considered the front-line screening method; some clinicians may opt to add a digital rectal exam.
3. Shared decision making with providers is key for individuals to make informed decisions about whether to undergo screening.
4. Screening should begin with a baseline PSA test between ages 40 and 45. Depending on health status, yearly PSA testing should be considered.
5. Individuals who have a family history of prostate cancer or high-risk genetic variants should consider starting screening at age 40.
6. After age 70, individuals should discuss with their provider whether to stop screening.

A recent increase in the incidence of men presenting with advanced prostate cancer has been attributed by some to the change in prostate cancer screening guidelines a decade ago, recommending against universal screening. The Prostate Cancer Foundation's stand-alone guideline for Black men provides evidence-based recommendations to lessen the burden of disease in this high-risk population.

- **Adverse Outcomes Following Curative Treatment for Prostate Cancer[61]**

*Functional outcomes at 10 years varied by type of treatment and prognosis*

Patients with clinically localized prostate cancer are typically offered an array of treatment options that may include active surveillance; radical prostatectomy; and radiotherapy, with or without androgen-deprivation therapy (ADT). No prospective data on disease outcomes provide support for either surgery or radiotherapy, therefore many patients make treatment decisions based on their understanding of the potential impact on urinary, sexual, or bowel function.

Investigators evaluated treatment-related functional outcomes in an observational study of 2,445 patients treated for localized prostate cancer who were enrolled in the Comparative Effectiveness Analysis of Surgery and Radiation (CEASAR) study. Patients were divided into two groups at the time of diagnosis: favorable prognosis (cT1 or T2a/bN0M0, prostate specific antigen (PSA) ≤20 ng/mL, and grade group 1–2) and unfavorable prognosis (cT2cN0M0, PSA 20–50 ng/mL, or grade group 3–5). The primary outcomes were 10-year patient reported sexual, urinary incontinence, urinary irritation, bowel, and hormone function domain scores, measured with the validated Prostate Cancer Index Composite (EPIC-26).

Patients' median age was 64 years. Patients in the favorable-prognosis group underwent radical prostatectomy (1088 patients), radiotherapy (380), active surveillance (414), and low-dose brachytherapy (96). Patients in the unfavorable-prognosis group underwent radical prostatectomy (387) and radiotherapy (220).

Among patients with favorable prognosis, those undergoing radical prostatectomy had worse urinary incontinence but no major difference in sexual function compared with patients followed with active surveillance. Among patients with unfavorable prognosis, those treated with radical prostatectomy had worse urinary incontinence but no major difference in sexual function compared with those treated with radiotherapy plus ADT; patients managed with radiotherapy plus ADT experienced worse bowel and hormone function than those treated with radical prostatectomy.

Patients faced with management decisions for clinically localized prostate cancer may seek out opinions from medical oncologists as neutral arbiters.

- **A Novel Inhibitor of Steroid-Hormone Biosynthesis in Advanced Prostate Cancer**[69]

*The agent showed antitumor activity in heavily pretreated patients in a phase 1/2 study.*

In a phase 1/2 trial, investigators evaluated ODM-208, a novel inhibitor of cytochrome P450 11A, in patients with progressive metastatic castration-resistant prostate cancer that had been treated with one or more androgen receptor pathway inhibitors and taxane-based chemotherapies. Phase 1 included 47 patients, regardless of androgen receptor (AR) gene mutation status, and phase 2 included 45 patients, all with AR mutations in plasma circulating tumor DNA.

In phase 2, the median age was 69 years, 84% of patients had received ≥3 lines of prior therapy, and 78% had Eastern Cooperative Oncology Group (ECOG) performance status 1. The most common mutation was L702H (41%). Patients were treated with ODM-208 (5 mg twice daily) plus dexamethasone (1 mg/day) and fludrocortisone (0.1 mg/day).

Prostate-specific antigen levels decreased by 50% or more in 73.7% of patients with AR mutations and 8.7% of patients with AR wild type in phase 1 and in 53.3% of patients (all with AR mutations) in phase 2.

The most-frequent treatment-emergent adverse event in phase 1 was adrenal insufficiency (36.2%). In phase 2, 80% of patients experienced grade ≥3 toxicity.

The trial demonstrated antitumor activity in a heavily treated population with AR mutations.

- **Results after Four Years of Screening for Prostate Cancer with PSA and MRI**[77]

*Systematic prostate biopsy and MRI versus MRI alone*

In this study involving over 13,000 men with a prostate-specific antigen (PSA) level of 3 ng/ml or higher, half were randomized to systematic prostate biopsy and magnetic resonance imaging (MRI) while the other half were randomized to MRI only. Repeat screening was performed at 2, 4 or 8 years later depending on their PSA level.

The number of advanced or high-risk cancers detected (by screening or as interval cancer) was 15 in the MRI-targeted biopsy group and 23 in the systematic biopsy group (relative risk, 0.65; 95% CI, 0.34 to 1.24). Five severe adverse events occurred, three in the systematic biopsy group and two in the MRI-targeted biopsy group).

The investigators concluded that omitting biopsy in patients with negative MRI results eliminated more than half of diagnoses of clinically insignificant prostate cancer, and the associated risk of having incurable cancer diagnosed at screening or as interval cancer was very low.

- **Does Stereotactic Body Radiotherapy (SBRT) Offer Benefit in Localized Prostate Cancer?[105]**

*Five-fraction SBRT was noninferior to standard radiotherapy for freedom from biochemical/clinical failure in patients with low- to intermediate-risk disease.*

5-fraction stereotactic body radiotherapy (SBRT) involves administering higher biologic doses per treatment session in fewer total sessions with the goal of reducing therapy-related toxicity while maintaining efficacy.

Investigators conducted an open-label, randomized, phase 3, noninferiority trial in men with clinical stage T1/T2 prostate cancer with a Gleason score of 3+4 or less and who had prostate-specific antigen (PSA) values ≤20 ng/mL. Participants received standard-of-care radiotherapy (using one of two standard treatment regimens) or SBRT in 5 fractions. No patients in either group received androgen deprivation therapy. The primary endpoint was freedom from biochemical (PSA) or clinical failure.

The findings were:

- At a median follow-up of 74 months, SBRT was noninferior to control radiotherapy; 5-year incidence of freedom from biochemical/clinical failure was 95.8% with SBRT and 94.6% with control radiotherapy.
- The incidence of late Radiation Therapy Oncology Group (RTOG) grade 2 or higher genitourinary and gastrointestinal toxic effects were 26.9% and 10.7%, respectively, with SBRT and 18.3% and 10.2% with control radiotherapy.

- **Transrectal versus Transperineal Prostate Biopsy[106]**

*In a randomized trial, procedure-related infection was less common with the transperineal approach.*

This U.S. multicenter randomized trial involved 742 men with elevated prostate-specific antigen (PSA) levels or palpable prostate abnormalities who were scheduled for prostate biopsy under local anesthesia. Patients underwent either transrectal biopsy (with antibiotic prophylaxis) or transperineal biopsy (without antibiotic prophylaxis). The primary outcome, infection after biopsy, occurred in fewer patients in the transperineal group than in the transrectal group (0 vs. 6 infections; p=0.02). The proportion of patients whose biopsies revealed prostate cancer was similar in the two groups.

- **$^{177}$Lu-PSMA-617 or a Change of androgen-receptor pathway inhibitor (ARPI) for Taxane-Naive Metastatic Castration-Resistant Prostate Cancer?[107]**

*$^{177}$Lu-PSMA-617 improved radiographic progression-free survival compared to a change in androgen-receptor pathway inhibitor.*

$^{177}$Lu-PSMA-617 is a prostate-specific membrane antigen (PSMA)–targeted radioligand therapy that is FDA approved for PSMA-positive, metastatic castration-resistant prostate cancer (mCRPC) with disease progression following treatment with an androgen-receptor pathway inhibitor (ARPI) and docetaxel. In a multinational, phase 3 trial, 468 patients with progressive docetaxel-naive mCRPC were randomized to switch to an alternative ARPI (abiraterone or enzalutamide) or to receive $^{177}$Lu-PSMA-617 once every 6 weeks for 6 cycles.

The findings were:

1. Radiographic progression-free survival, the primary outcome, was significantly improved in the $^{177}$Lu-PSMA-617 arm compared to the alternative-ARPI arm (median, 11.6 vs. 5.6 months).
2. Grade 3–5 adverse events were less frequent with $^{177}$Lu-PSMA-617 than with the alternative ARPI (36% vs. 48%)
3. Overall survival did not differ between groups.

## CHAPTER 6. RENAL CANCER

- **Novel Radiotracer PET-CT Imaging: A Non-invasive Method to Characterize Small Renal Masses**[89]

*PET-CT imaging using [$^{89}$Zr] Zr-girentuximab, a radiolabeled monoclonal antibody that binds to an antigen expressed on tumor cells, was found to be highly sensitive and specific for detecting clear-cell renal carcinoma*

The investigators conducted an open-label, multicenter, phase 3 trial of positron-emission tomography (PET)–CT imaging using [$^{89}$Zr] Zr-girentuximab, a chimeric monoclonal antibody directed against an antigen associated with renal cell carcinoma (RCC), to determine its sensitivity and specificity in detecting clear-cell renal cell carcinoma. A single dose of [$^{89}$Zr] Zr-girentuximab followed by PET-CT was administered to 332 patients with evidence of a solitary, localized indeterminate renal mass ≤7 cm suspicious for renal cell carcinoma who were scheduled for nephrectomy.

The mean sensitivity of [$^{89}$Zr] Zr-girentuximab PET-CT imaging was 85.5% and the specificity was 87.0%.

Urologists who currently manage patients with suspected RCC use lesion size, characteristics, and rate of change on CT/MRI to make therapy recommendations, with tissue confirmation required for interventions. Thus, this technique appears a useful addition to the diagnostic work-up of RCC, although it should be noted that all PET-positive lesions in this study were malignant.

- **Combination Anti–PD-1 Therapy and VEGFR TKI in Heavily Treated Advanced Renal Cell Cancer[91]**

*This study provides evidence that the combination of anti–PD-1 therapy plus vascular endothelial growth factor receptor (VEGFR) tyrosine kinase inhibitors (TKIs) should not be routinely used for renal cell carcinoma refractory to immune checkpoint inhibitors.*

In this study the investigators randomized 343 patients with metastatic clear-cell renal cancer with disease progression following 1 or 2 prior therapies (including one immune checkpoint inhibitor (ICI) to receive tivozanib, a selective VEGFR tyrosine kinase inhibitor (TKI), either alone or in combination with nivolumab, a PD-1 checkpoint inhibitor. During a median follow-up of 12 months, the primary endpoint of progression-free survival (PFS) was not significantly different between treatment arms (median PFS, 7.4 months for tivozanib alone vs. 5.7 months for tivozanib/nivolumab).

- **Salvage Therapy for Advanced Clear-Cell Renal Cancer[97]**

*Patients with progressive renal cell carcinoma following immune checkpoint and antiangiogenic therapies had better progression-free survival with the HIF-2α inhibitor belzutifan than with everolimus.*

For patients with progressive, metastatic clear-cell renal cancer after treatment with immune checkpoint inhibitors (ICIs) and vascular endothelial growth factor receptor–tyrosine kinase inhibitors (VEGFR-TKIs), effective management options are limited. Alteration of the VHL gene occurs in the majority of clear-cell renal cancers and is associated with dysregulation of the hypoxia-inducible factor (HIF) pathway as a consequence of accumulation of HIF-2α. Belzutifan is a small-molecule inhibitor of HIF-2α with demonstrated activity in clear-cell renal cancer.

The investigators performed a phase 3 trial of 746 patients with advanced clear-cell renal cancer previously treated with ICIs and antiangiogenic agents in which patients were randomized to receive either belzutifan (120 mg daily) or everolimus (10 mg daily).

Most patients (86%) had received two or three previous lines of therapy. At a median follow-up of 18.4 months, although the median PFS was 5.6 months in both arms, significantly more patients in the belzutifan arm than the everolimus arm were alive and free of progression (24% vs. 8.3%; p=0.002). At a median follow-up of 25.7 months, the median OS did not differ significantly between arms.

## CHAPTER 7. MELANOMA

- **Final Results from a Study of Adjuvant Therapy in Stage III Melanoma[9]**

*A predefined subset analysis of patients with the most common mutation (V600E) suggested a 25% OS benefit with dabrafenib/trametinib. In contrast, in patients with the less common V600K mutation, OS appeared to be inferior in those treated with dabrafenib/trametinib compared with placebo.*

In this study researchers report the final results from the COMBI-AD trail, in which 870 patients with resected stage III melanoma with *BRAF* mutations were randomized to adjuvant dabrafenib plus trametinib or placebo for 1 year. At approximately 8 years of follow-up, there was a nonsignificant trend towards better overall survival (OS) in the dabrafenib/trametinib group compared with the placebo group (71% vs. 65%; ratio for death, 0.80; *p*=0.06). A predefined subset analysis of patients with the most common mutation (*V600E*) suggested a 25% OS benefit with dabrafenib/trametinib. In contrast, in patients with the less common *V600K* mutation, OS appeared to be inferior in those treated with dabrafenib/trametinib compared with placebo (HR, 1.95).

- **Neoadjuvant Treatment Takes Center Stage for Patients with Resectable Melanoma[11]**

*The combination of nivolumab and ipilimumab before surgery yielded better event-free survival but greater toxicity than nivolumab after surgery.*

In the NADINA trial researchers compared outcomes of 423 patients assigned either to two doses of neoadjuvant treatment (nivolumab plus ipilimumab) before surgery or to surgery upfront followed by adjuvant nivolumab alone (≤12 cycles).

Patients in the neoadjuvant arm who had a major pathologic response (59%) were given no further systemic therapy; those who had a pathologic partial response (8%) or nonresponse (26%) received adjuvant nivolumab or combination dabrafenib/trametinib. Estimated 12-month event-free survival was significantly superior in the neoadjuvant arm, compared with the adjuvant arm (84% vs. 57%). The neoadjuvant regimen was associated with a higher rate of systemic-treatment–related grade ≥3 adverse events (30% vs. 15% in the adjuvant arm).

- **A Neoantigen Vaccine for Melanoma?**[62]

*Results from a randomized trial make a compelling argument that cancer vaccines warrant further investigation.*

Investigators presented results from the phase 2b KEYNOTE-942 trial, the first randomized study of a neoantigen vaccine plus pembrolizumab with a clinical efficacy endpoint.

Using new technology in the form of an mRNA vaccine, researchers created a platform to deliver a unique, personalized, cancer-specific neoantigen vaccine (mRNA-4157 [V940]) based on each patients' individual cancer mutations. In the open-label, randomized (2:1) study of 157 patients with high-risk, resected stage III or IV melanoma, those who received the combination of this neoantigen vaccine and pembrolizumab were more likely to be free from recurrent melanoma at 18 months than those who received pembrolizumab alone (79% vs. 62%; two-sided $p$=0.053). There were no grade 4–5 adverse events associated with the neoantigen vaccine.

- **Final 10-Year Outcomes with Nivolumab plus Ipilimumab in Advanced Melanoma[87]**

*The final trial results showed a continued, ongoing survival benefit with nivolumab plus ipilimumab and with nivolumab monotherapy, as compared with ipilimumab monotherapy, in patients with advanced melanoma.*

In this trial, patients with previously untreated advanced melanoma were randomized in a 1:1:1 ratio, to one of the following regimens:

1. Nivolumab (1 mg per kilogram of body weight) plus ipilimumab (3 mg per kilogram) every 3 weeks for four doses, followed by nivolumab (3 mg per kilogram) every 2 weeks
2. Nivolumab (3 mg per kilogram) every 2 weeks plus placebo
3. Ipilimumab (3 mg per kilogram) every 3 weeks for four doses plus placebo.

Treatment was continued until the occurrence of disease progression, unacceptable toxic effects, or withdrawal of consent. Randomization was stratified according to *BRAF* mutation status, metastasis stage, and programmed death ligand 1 (PDL-1) expression.

With a minimum follow-up of 10 years, median overall survival was 71.9 months with nivolumab plus ipilimumab, 36.9 months with nivolumab, and 19.9 months with ipilimumab. The hazard ratio for death was 0.53 for nivolumab plus ipilimumab compared with ipilimumab and was 0.63 for nivolumab compared with ipilimumab. Median melanoma-specific survival was more than 120 months with nivolumab plus ipilimumab, 49.4 months with nivolumab, and 21.9 months with ipilimumab.

Among patients who had been alive and progression-free at 3 years, 10-year melanoma-specific survival was 96% with nivolumab plus ipilimumab, 97% with nivolumab, and 88% with ipilimumab.

This study emphasizes the extraordinary improvement in outcome for patients with advanced melanoma due to the introduction of checkpoint inhibitors. These agents suppress the suppression of the immune system induced by the tumours themselves. It also illustrates that the use of combination checkpoint inhibitors – each targeting a different inhibitor – appears superior to using a single checkpoint inhibitor – echoing the pattern seen with combination cytotoxic chemotherapy.

It is of interest that checkpoint inhibitors have been especially beneficial in melanoma – a tumor that is known to be particularly susceptible to control by a normally functioning immune system

## Chapter 8. PANCREATIC CANCER

- **Nimotuzumab May Effectively Target *KRAS* Wild-Type Pancreatic Cancer[42]**

*The addition of the EGFR-targeting monoclonal antibody nimotuzumab to gemcitabine improved progression-free survival in this subset of patients.*

The epidermal growth factor receptor (EGFR)–targeted tyrosine kinase inhibitor gefitinib is FDA-approved in combination with gemcitabine in metastatic pancreatic cancer. However, the benefits are marginal. Mutations in *KRAS*, which are present in nearly 90% of pancreatic cancers, may obtain benefit from EGFR-targeted agents.

In this study investigators reported results of a randomized, placebo-controlled trial in patients with *KRAS* wild-type advanced pancreatic cancer who had received no prior chemotherapy for metastatic disease. Patients received either

1. Weekly gemcitabine for 3 weeks on and 1 week off combined with either placebo or the EGFR-targeting monoclonal antibody nimotuzumab given weekly.
   or
2. Nimotuzumab given weekly.

Of 480 patients screened for *KRAS* wild-type status, 82 (17%) were identified; median age was 55, 56% had undergone prior surgery, and 7% had received prior adjuvant chemotherapy.

The primary endpoint of overall survival (OS) trended higher with nimotuzumab compared with placebo (median, 10.9 vs. 8.5 months; hazard ratio, 0.66; *p*=0.08). Progression-free survival was longer with nimotuzumab compared with placebo (median, 4.2 vs. 3.6 months; HR, 0.60; *P*=0.04). Rates of response (7.3% and. 9.8%) and disease control (63.4% and 68.3%) were similar between treatment arms. Rates of adverse events were also similar between the two arms.

This trial targeting the subset of patients with *KRAS* wild-type pancreatic cancer indicates activity for an EGFR-targeting antibody. Further study of EGFR-targeted therapies in *KRAS* wild-type pancreatic cancer is warranted.

- **Novel Sequenced Chemotherapy Regimen for Metastatic Pancreatic Cancer[44]**

*Treatment with gemcitabine plus nab-paclitaxel followed by mFOLFOX was associated with higher survival and response rate than treatment with gemcitabine plus nab-paclitaxel alone.*

The optimal first-line chemotherapy for advanced pancreatic cancer, validated in phase 3 trials, is the triplet combination of infusional 5-FU, oxaliplatin, and either irinotecan or nanoliposome-encapsulated irinotecan (FOLFIRINOX or NALIRIFOX). Now, in a randomized, phase 2 trial involving patients with metastatic pancreatic cancer, investigators compared the combination of gemcitabine and *nab*-paclitaxel to a novel sequenced regimen of gemcitabine and *nab*-paclitaxel followed by mFOLFOX-6 on a 6-week cycle. *Nab*-paclitaxel is paclitaxel combined with albumin

Of 157 patients, the median age was 66, 94% had metastatic disease, only 18% had undergone prior surgery, and 4% had received prior chemotherapy. The primary endpoint of 12-month overall survival (OS) was higher with the sequenced regimen compared with gemcitabine/*nab*-paclitaxel alone (55.3% vs. 35.4%, *P*=0.02); median OS was also higher (13.2 vs. 9.7 months; hazard ratio, 0.68). Median progression-free survival was higher with the sequenced regimen (7.0 vs 5.2 months; HR, 0.52) as was the response rate (39.7% vs. 20.3%). Adverse events and rates of grade 3/4 neurologic toxicity were similar between the two treatment arms.

This small phase 2 trial indicates potential superiority for the sequencing of mFOLFOX6 with gemcitabine/*nab*-paclitaxel compared with gemcitabine/*nab*-paclitaxel alone. However, this sequencing regimen offers no clear advantage over the two approved triplet regimens, FOLFIRINOX and NALIRIFOX.

## CHAPTER 9. HEAD AND NECK CANCER

- Induction-concurrent chemoradiotherapy with or without sintilimab in patients with locoregionally advanced nasopharyngeal carcinoma[5]

*The addition of the anti-PD1 antibody sintilimab to chemoradiotherapy reduced distant metastasis and locoregional recurrence in patients with locoregionally advanced EBV-positive nasopharynx cancer (NPC)*

425 patients with NPC were randomized to induction gemcitabine and cisplatin followed by definitive concurrent chemoradiotherapy either with or without the addition of sintilimab (200 mg once every 3 weeks for 12 cycles). At a median follow-up of 42 months, event-free survival, the primary outcome, was superior in the sintilimab group compared to the control group (3-year event-free survival rate, 86% vs. 76%; hazard ratio, 0.59). The sintilimab group also showed significantly improved distant metastasis-free survival (90% vs. 83%) and locoregional recurrence-free survival (93% vs. 86%) at 3 years, but overall survival did not differ between groups (92% in both). However, grade ≥3 immune-related adverse events, including two deaths, occurred in 11% of the sintilimab group versus none in the control group.

- **Tumor Hypoxia-Directed De-Escalation of Chemoradiotherapy for Locally Advanced HPV-Related Oropharyngeal Carcinoma[58]**

*Patients without tumor hypoxia as assessed by $^{18}$F-fluoromisonidazole PET had promising survival outcomes after treatment with reduced-dose radiation and chemotherapy.*

Human papillomavirus (HPV)–related oropharyngeal carcinoma has excellent prognosis when treated with standard chemoradiotherapy, but this can cause significant toxicity. De-escalation of standard therapy has been attempted in many clinical trials with various strategies, yet none has demonstrated noninferiority in a phase 3 randomized clinical trial. Tumor hypoxia has been associated with radiation resistance.

To assess whether measurement of tumor hypoxia could identify candidates for de-escalation of chemoradiotherapy, investigators enrolled 152 patients with HPV-related oropharyngeal cancer with stage T0-2/N1-2c/M0 disease in a single-arm, single-center, phase 2 study.

Patients underwent primary tumor resection followed by baseline $^{18}$F-fluoromisonidazole (FMISO) positron emission tomography (PET) scan to determine tumor hypoxia. Those with hypoxia had repeat FMISO PET 1 to 2 weeks intratreatment. Patients with no hypoxia at baseline (n=42) or hypoxia resolution during treatment (n=86) received a total of 30 Gy of radiation and 2 cycles of chemotherapy (cisplatin 100 mg/m$^2$ or carboplatin AUC=5 and 5-FU 2400 mg/m$^2$ over 4 days). Patients with baseline or persistent hypoxia (n=24) received a total of 70 Gy of radiation and 3 cycles of chemotherapy.

Progression-free survival (PFS) at 2 years was similar in the 30-Gy and 70-Gy cohorts (94% and 96%), while the 30-Gy cohort had significantly lower rates of acute and late grade 3 and 4 adverse events (acute, 32% vs. 58.3%; late, 0% vs. 4.5%, respectively).

De-escalation approaches for HPV-related head and neck cancer have shown promising results, with reduced adverse events and improved quality of life, but have not yet demonstrated noninferiority to standard chemoradiotherapy. Although the current study demonstrated promising PFS for patients with no tumor hypoxia at baseline or hypoxia that resolved early on-treatment who received 30-Gy radiation and chemotherapy, this approach remains investigational and needs to be validated in a phase 3 randomized clinical trial.

- **Adding an Immune Checkpoint Inhibitor to Standard Treatment for EBV-Positive Nasopharynx Cancer[104]**

*Another study showing the benefit of adding sintilimab to chemotherapy in EBV-positive nasopharyngeal cancer:*

*The addition of the anti-PD1 antibody sintilimab to chemoradiotherapy reduced distant metastasis and locoregional recurrence in patients with locoregionally advanced EBV-positive nasopharynx cancer.*

In a multicenter, open-label, randomized, controlled, phase 3 study conducted in China, researchers evaluated the anti-PD1 antibody sintilimab; 425 patients with NPC were randomized to induction gemcitabine and cisplatin followed by definitive concurrent chemoradiotherapy either with or without the addition of sintilimab (200 mg once every 3 weeks for 12 cycles). At a median follow-up of 42 months, event-free survival, the primary outcome, was superior in the sintilimab group compared with the control group (3-year rate, 86% vs. 76%; hazard ratio, 0.59). The sintilimab group had significantly improved distant metastasis-free survival (90% vs. 83%) and locoregional recurrence-free survival (93% vs. 86%) at 3 years, but overall survival did not differ between groups (92% in both).

Grade 3–4 adverse events were more frequent in the sintilimab group (74% vs. 65%); both groups experienced similar rates of mucositis, cytopenia, nausea, and vomiting, but grade ≥3 immune-related adverse events, including two deaths, occurred in 11% of the sintilimab group versus none in the control group.

## CHAPTER 10. UROTHELIAL CANCER

- **Paradigm Shift in the Management of Advanced Urothelial Cancer[47]**

*Compared with platinum-based chemotherapy, enfortumab vedotin plus pembrolizumab treatment led to better survival outcomes in patients with previously untreated advanced urothelial cancer.*

Platinum-based chemotherapy has long been the standard of care for metastatic urothelial cancer, with cisplatin eligibility determined based on clinical and laboratory features. Recently, both pembrolizumab, a PD-1 inhibitor, and enfortumab vedotin, an antibody–drug conjugate directed against nectin-4, demonstrated improved overall survival (OS) compared with a variety of chemotherapeutic agents in phase 3 studies, and the combination of enfortumab vedotin and pembrolizumab (EVP) demonstrated antitumor activity in a phase 2 study.

Now, in a global, phase 3, randomized trial, investigators compared platinum-based chemotherapy (gemcitabine plus cisplatin or carboplatin) against EVP.

Eligible patients had unresectable or metastatic urothelial cancer with adequate organ function and performance status (ECOG score ≤2). Perioperative chemotherapy was permitted if recurrence occurred more than 1 year after completion of therapy. Of 886 patients, the median age was 69 and most were male (77%) and white (68%); <2% were African-American.

At a median follow-up of 17.2 months, the two primary outcomes — progression-free survival (PFS) and overall survival (OS) — were longer in the EVP group than the chemotherapy group (median PFS, 12.5 vs. 6.3 months; hazard ratio, 0.45; $p<$ 0.001; and median OS, 31.5 vs. 16.1 months; HR, 0.47; $p<$ 0.001). Any grade neuropathy occurred in 50.0% of patients in the EVP group and led to discontinuation of treatment in 10.7%. Grade 3 or higher treatment-related adverse events occurred in 55.9% of the EVP group and 69.5% of the chemotherapy group, most commonly maculopapular rash (7.7%), hyperglycemia (5.0%), and neutropenia (4.8%) with EVP and anemia (31.4%), neutropenia (30.0%), and thrombocytopenia (19.4%) with chemotherapy.

The EVP regimen had a challenging side-effect profile, including neuropathy and skin toxicity, that required close patient monitoring.

- **Adjuvant Pembrolizumab versus Observation in Muscle-Invasive Urothelial Carcinoma**[85]

*Among patients with high-risk muscle-invasive urothelial carcinoma after radical surgery, disease-free survival was significantly longer with adjuvant pembrolizumab than with observation.*

In a phase 3 trial, investigators randomly assigned patients, who had undergone radical surgery for muscle-invasive urothelial cancer, in a 1:1 ratio, to receive pembrolizumab at a dose of 200 mg every 3 weeks for 1 year or to undergo observation. Randomization was stratified according to pathological stage, centrally tested programmed death ligand 1 (PD-L1) status, and previous neoadjuvant chemotherapy.

With a median duration of follow-up for disease-free survival of 44.8 months, the median disease-free survival was 29.6 months with pembrolizumab and 14.2 months with observation (p-value = 0.003).

- **Perioperative Durvalumab with Neoadjuvant Chemotherapy in Operable Bladder Cancer[80]**

*Perioperative durvalumab plus neoadjuvant chemotherapy led to significant improvements in event-free survival and overall survival in muscle-invasive bladder cancer compared with neoadjuvant chemotherapy alone.*

Neoadjuvant chemotherapy with cisplatin and gemcitabine followed by radical cystectomy is the standard treatment for cisplatin-eligible patients with muscle-invasive bladder cancer. In this phase 3 randomized clinical trial the investigators explored whether the addition of durvalumab, an immune checkpoint inhibitor, would improve outcome.

The estimated event-free survival at 24 months was 67.8% in the durvalumab group and 59.8% in the comparison group (p<0.001). The estimated overall survival at 24 months was 82.2% in the durvalumab group and 75.2% in the comparison group (p=0.01). Grade 3 or 4 treatment-related adverse events was similar between the two groups

- **Does Adding Pembrolizumab to Chemoradiotherapy Improve Survival in Patients with Locally Advanced Cervical Cancer?[34]**

*The addition of pembrolizumab to standard chemoradiotherapy followed by pembrolizumab maintenance improved progression-free survival compared with chemoradiotherapy alone.*

Using pembrolizumab with platinum-based chemotherapy has been shown to be effective in patients with PD-L1–positive, persistent, recurrent, or metastatic cervical cancer. In a randomized, double-blind, international, phase 3 trial, researchers evaluated survival outcomes with pembrolizumab in 1,060 adult patients with locally advanced cervical cancer who were receiving chemoradiation.

Eligible patients had newly diagnosed, high-risk squamous cell carcinoma, adenocarcinoma, or adenosquamous carcinoma of the cervix (FIGO 2014 stage IB2–IIB with node-positive disease or stage III–IVA). The study arms were either pembrolizumab plus chemoradiotherapy followed by maintenance pembrolizumab, *or* placebo plus chemoradiotherapy followed by maintenance placebo. Over 94% of study participants had positive PD-L1 expression (combined positive score, ≥1). (FIGO is the abbreviation for the Federation of Gynecology and Obstetrics).

The median follow-up was almost 18 months in both arms. Rates of progression-free survival at 24 months were 68% in the pembrolizumab arm and 57% in the placebo arm, with a hazard ratio for disease progression or death of 0.70, a significant finding. Estimated overall survival at 24 months was 87% in the pembrolizumab arm and 81% in the placebo arm. A higher percentage of patients in the pembrolizumab arm than in the placebo arm experienced grade 3 or higher adverse events (75% and 69%, respectively), but no new safety signals were identified.

These results suggest a role for pembrolizumab in the treatment of locally advanced cervical cancer in combination with chemoradiotherapy and as maintenance therapy.

- **Is Simple Hysterectomy Noninferior to Radical Hysterectomy in Low-Risk Cervical Cancer?[50]**

*In carefully selected patients with lesions ≤2 cm and low-risk features, simple hysterectomy was not inferior to radical hysterectomy.*

Radical hysterectomy is the standard of care for women with a diagnosis of early-stage cervical cancer, but this surgery is known to a have higher risk of perioperative complications than a more-conservative surgical procedure. In an international trial investigators assessed whether simple hysterectomy is noninferior to radical hysterectomy in patients with early-stage cervical cancer and low-risk features.

Eligibility criteria included squamous cell carcinoma, adenocarcinoma, or adenosquamous carcinoma histologies of any grade; FIGO stage IA2 or IB1 (lesion ≤2 cm); limited stromal invasion; and no evidence of lymph node involvement on preoperative imaging. A total of 700 patients were randomized to either radical hysterectomy or simple hysterectomy; however, the surgical approach (open vs. minimally invasive) was at the discretion of the trial surgeons and was not a stratification factor. Most patients (92%) had stage IB1 disease.

The incidence of pelvic recurrence at 3 years (the primary outcome) was 2.52% in the simple hysterectomy arm and 2.17% in the radical hysterectomy arm. Simple hysterectomy was not inferior to radical hysterectomy. Simple hysterectomy was also associated with significantly lower rates of urinary retention and incontinence.

In carefully selected patients with early stage, low-risk cervical cancer, simple hysterectomy may be considered as an alternative to radical hysterectomy.

- **Tisotumab Vedotin as Second- or Third-Line Therapy for Recurrent Cervical Cancer[75]**

*Median overall survival was significantly longer in the tisotumab vedotin group than in the chemotherapy group*

Investigators conducted a phase 3, multinational, open-label trial of tisotumab vedotin as second- or third-line therapy in patients with recurrent or metastatic cervical cancer. Patients were randomly assigned, in a 1:1 ratio, to receive tisotumab vedotin monotherapy (2.0 mg per kilogram of body weight every 3 weeks) or the investigator's choice of chemotherapy (topotecan, vinorelbine, gemcitabine, irinotecan, or pemetrexed). The primary end point was overall survival.

Tisotumab vedotin is a combination of tisotumab, a monoclonal antibody against tissue factor, and monomethyl auristatin E, a potent inhibitor of cell division.

A total of 502 patients underwent randomization (253 were assigned to the tisotumab vedotin group and 249 to the chemotherapy group); the groups were similar with respect to demographic and disease characteristics. The median overall survival was significantly longer in the tisotumab vedotin group than in the chemotherapy group (11.5 months vs. 9.5 months [95% CI, 7.9 to 10.7]), results that represented a 30% lower risk of death with tisotumab vedotin than with chemotherapy (hazard ratio, 0.70; two-sided p=0.004). The median progression-free survival was 4.2 months (95% CI, 4.0 to 4.4) with tisotumab vedotin and 2.9 months (95% CI, 2.6 to 3.1) with chemotherapy (hazard ratio, 0.67; 95% CI, 0.54 to 0.82; two-sided P<0.001). The confirmed objective response rate was 17.8% in the tisotumab vedotin group and 5.2% in the chemotherapy group (odds ratio, 4.0; two-sided p<0.001).

A total of 98.4% of patients in the tisotumab vedotin group and 99.2% in the chemotherapy group had at least one adverse event that occurred during the treatment period (defined as the period from day 1 of dose 1 until 30 days after the last dose); grade 3 or greater events occurred in 52.0% and 62.3%, respectively. A total of 14.8% of patients stopped tisotumab vedotin treatment because of toxic effects.

In patients with recurrent cervical cancer, second- or third-line treatment with tisotumab vedotin resulted in significantly greater efficacy than chemotherapy.

- **Adding an Immune Checkpoint Inhibitor to BRAF/MEK Inhibitors for *BRAF* V600E-Mutated Anaplastic Thyroid Cancer[35]**

*Adding pembrolizumab to combined dabrafenib and trametinib shows a promising improvement in patients' overall survival in a retrospective, single-center study.*

Anaplastic thyroid carcinoma is an aggressive cancer, with the *BRAF* V600E mutation driving approximately 40% of cases. The FDA has approved the combination of the BRAF inhibitor dabrafenib with the MEK inhibitor trametinib (DT) for patients with this disease. Despite the combination's overall response rate (ORR) of 69%, updated analyses reveal an ORR of 56% and a median overall survival (OS) of 14.5 months, indicating limited long-term benefits. To investigate whether adding an immune checkpoint inhibitor enhances the durability of response, researchers in this study retrospectively examined the effect of pembrolizumab.

In the dataset, 23 patients with anaplastic thyroid carcinoma were treated with DT, and 48 received DT combined with pembrolizumab (DTP). Median OS was significantly longer in the DTP group compared to the DT group (17 months vs. 9 months), although the ORR was similar in the groups (64.5% and 73.3%, respectively). In the DTP group, 14 patients received pembrolizumab at progression, and 34 received upfront DTP, but the median OS did not differ between these patient subgroups (16 and 17 months, respectively). In a separate group of 23 patients, presurgical DTP was linked to a 50% pathological complete response rate and a median OS of 63 months. Safety profiles were acceptable, with immune-related adverse events observed in 32% of patients, none of which were grade 5.

Although DT has revolutionized the treatment of patients with *BRAF* V600E-mutated anaplastic thyroid carcinoma, the combination's durability is limited. In these authors' experience, adding pembrolizumab to DT significantly prolonged OS. Neoadjuvant DTP was linked to impressive pathological complete response rates and prolonged median OS. These results suggest that combining an immune checkpoint inhibitor with BRAF/MEK inhibitors can extend survival in patients with *BRAF* V600E-mutated anaplastic thyroid carcinoma, although further validation, including phase 3 randomized clinical trials, is warranted.

- **Initial Treatment of *BRAF* V600E-Variant Anaplastic Thyroid Cancer[90]**

*This consensus statement presents clinical practice standards and recommendations from a multidisciplinary team at a large academic cancer center. The statement does not contradict the current guidelines from the American Thyroid Association and the National Comprehensive Cancer Network, but it does describe a complex treatment pathway that most likely requires multidisciplinary care.*

A new consensus statement on treatment and management of *BRAF* V600E-mutated anaplastic thyroid cancer (ATC) emphasizes rapid identification of *BRAF* status by immunohistochemistry or polymerase chain reaction followed by timely initiation of systemic therapy. The Thyroid Neck Morbidity Complexity (TNMC) score is used to determine whether neoadjuvant treatment is needed. The proposed algorithm for initial management of stage IVb ATC involves neoadjuvant dabrafenib with the MEK inhibitor trametinib (DT) or pembrolizumab + DT (DTP) for patients with unresectable or advanced disease (TNMC ≥1), while patients without radiographic evidence of extrathyroidal or extranodal extension (TNMC 0) should proceed with upfront surgery.

In this report the authors authors favored DTP over DT, as it was associated with better overall survival, but the addition of pembrolizumab can be delayed, as the extent of tumor shrinkage is mainly dependent on the use of DT. After 2 to 3 months of neoadjuvant therapy, patients should be reassessed for resectability with contrast-enhanced computed tomography or PET/CT, and then treated surgically if feasible. DT(P) should be withheld during adjuvant chemoradiation, but can be resumed after completion of radiation.

For stage IVc ATC with distant metastasis, once brain metastasis is ruled out, the authors recommended starting DTP. Patients should also be considered for surgery if the disease is resectable after 2 to 3 months of systemic therapy. Complete resection of the primary tumor should be considered because it improves the quality of life, prevents complications, and prolongs survival even in patients with distant metastases.

## CHAPTER 13. GASTRIC CANCER

- **A new treatment option for advanced gastric cancer or gastro-oesophageal cancer?[8]**

*Overall survival was improved with tislelizumab over placebo*

Investigators reported the results of a multinational, industry-sponsored, placebo-controlled randomized trial comparing investigators' choice of first-line chemotherapy (capecitabine/oxaliplatin or infusional 5-FU/cisplatin) with or without the addition of the anti–PD-1 agent tislelizumab (200 mg every 3 weeks). Of the 997 patients enrolled, 75% were treated in Asia, 38% had liver metastases, 44% had peritoneal metastases, 80% had gastric primary tumors, and 4% had microsatellite instability (MSI)–high or DNA mismatch repair protein–deficient tumors. PDL-1 expression by tumor area positivity (TAP) combining tumor and immune cell staining was ≥5% in 55% and <5% in 45% of patients.

The primary endpoint of OS was improved with tislelizumab compared to placebo in patients with TAP ≥5% (median, 17.2% vs. 12.6 months; hazard ratio, 0.74; P=0.006); PFS was also significantly improved (HR, 0.67), and response rate was numerically improved. Among all treated patients, OS was also improved with tislelizumab over placebo (median, 15.0 vs. 12.9 months; HR, 0.80; p=0.001). The OS benefit for tislelizumab over placebo was diminished in patients with TAP <5% (HR, 0.92; 95% confidence limits, 0.75–1.13).

- **Neoadjuvant and Adjuvant Pembrolizumab in Locally Advanced Gastric Cancer or Gastro-oesophageal cancer[111]**

*The addition of pembrolizumab to chemotherapy improved response but not event-free survival.*

Immune checkpoint inhibitors improve response, progression-free survival, and overall survival when added to first-line chemotherapy in patients with esophagogastric adenocarcinoma. Investigators now report results of KEYNOTE-585, an international, phase 3 trial evaluating the addition of pembrolizumab to pre- and postoperative chemotherapy in patients with clinical stage T3–4 or node-positive resectable gastric cancer.

A main cohort of 804 patients were randomized to receive either pembrolizumab (200 mg) or placebo combined with chemotherapy — investigator's choice of capecitabine plus cisplatin or a 5-day infusion of fluorouracil (FU) plus cisplatin — for 3 cycles before surgery and 3 cycles after, followed by 11 cycles of placebo or pembrolizumab.

Another cohort of 203 patients were randomized to receive pembrolizumab or placebo combined with an alternative chemotherapy regimen of 5-FU, oxaliplatin, and docetaxel (FLOT) for 4 cycles pre- and 4 cycles post-surgery. In the main cohort 79% had gastric primary tumors, 75% had PD-L1 combined positive scores ≥1%, 9% had microsatellite instability (MSI)- high status, and 76% had clinical stage III disease.

The primary endpoint of pathologic complete response was improved with pembrolizumab compared with placebo in the main cohort (12.9% vs. 2.0%; $p<0.00001$) and in the combined main cohort plus FLOT cohort (13.0% vs. 2.4%). A co-primary endpoint of event-free survival was not significantly improved with pembrolizumab compared with placebo (hazard ratio, 0.81), despite numeric superiority for pembrolizumab (median, 44.4 vs. 25.3 months); results were similar in the combined cohort (45.8 vs 25.7 months). There was no difference in overall survival between the pembrolizumab and placebo arms in the main cohort (median, 60.7 vs. 58.0 months; HR, 0.90; $p=0.174$) or the combined cohort (median, 60.7 vs. 45.7 months).

Despite an improved rate of pathologic complete response with the addition of pembrolizumab to preoperative chemotherapy in patients with esophagogastric cancer, there were no significant improvements in event-free or overall survival.

- **New Estimates of Cancer Risk with Germline *CDH1* Variants**[72]

*In individuals carrying such variants, the lifetime risk of gastric cancer may be lower than previously thought, except in those with a strong family history of the disease.*

Germline pathogenic (P) or likely pathogenic (LP) loss-of-function variants in the *CDH1* gene are known to increase lifetime risks of gastric cancer and breast cancer, but the risk estimates to date (~50%) have been based on select populations, usually without consideration of the influence of cancer in other family members.

To better estimate these risks, researchers conducted a retrospective cohort study in North America involving 7,323 individuals from 213 families that had more than one family member with a P/LP *CDH1* variant. Genotyping was performed by certified diagnostic laboratories, with single-site analysis if a *CDH1* variant existed in the family, single *CDH1* gene analysis if personal and family history suggested hereditary diffuse gastric cancer, and multigene panel analysis if personal or family history overlapped with more than one syndrome.

Among individuals who carried a P/LP *CDH1* variant, the lifetime risk of advanced gastric cancer was 10% in men and 7% in women. The risk was substantially higher (38%) in carriers with a strong family history of gastric cancer (three affected first-degree relatives), suggesting that other genetic factors may also be at play. The lifetime risk of breast cancer among female carriers was 37%.

The estimated risk for breast cancer in this study is similar to previous estimates, but the estimated risk for gastric cancer is much lower. Limitations of the analysis include absence of complete clinical data, lack of information about the effects of risk-reducing surgery, and lack of information regarding ancestry and other potential familial factors affecting risk.

Current National Comprehensive Cancer Network guidelines recommend that individuals with P/LP variants of *CDH1* undergo annual screening mammograms and consider breast magnetic resonance imaging with and without contrast starting at age 30. The option of risk-reduction mastectomy should also be discussed. How best to manage gastric cancer risk in these individuals in the absence of a strong family history is unclear.

- **Preoperative Chemoradiotherapy for Resectable Gastric Cancer**[86]

*The addition of preoperative chemoradiotherapy to perioperative chemotherapy did not improve overall survival as compared with perioperative chemotherapy alone among patients with resectable gastric and gastroesophageal junction adenocarcinoma.*

In a phase 3 trial, patients with resectable adenocarcinoma of the stomach or gastroesophageal junction were randomly assigned to receive preoperative chemoradiotherapy plus perioperative chemotherapy or perioperative chemotherapy alone. In both groups, patients received either epirubicin, cisplatin, and fluorouracil or fluorouracil, leucovorin, oxaliplatin, and docetaxel both before and after surgery; the preoperative-chemoradiotherapy group also received chemoradiotherapy (45 Gy in 25 fractions of radiation, plus fluorouracil infusion).

A higher percentage of patients in the preoperative-chemoradiotherapy group than in the perioperative-chemotherapy group had a pathological complete response (17% vs. 8%) and greater tumor downstaging after resection. However, at a median follow-up of 67 months, no significant differences between the two groups for overall survival or progression-free survival were noted. The median overall survival was 46 months with preoperative chemoradiotherapy and 49 months with perioperative chemotherapy and the median progression-free survival was 31 months and 32 months, respectively.

- **Sintilimab Added to Chemotherapy for Advanced Esophagogastric Adenocarcinoma**[65]

*The addition of sintilimab improved outcomes, particularly in patients with combined positive scores (CPS) for PDL-1 >5%.*

Immune checkpoint inhibitors targeting PD-1 have been shown to improve response, progression-free survival, and overall survival when combined with first-line chemotherapy in patients with metastatic esophagogastric cancer. Investigators in China now report results of ORIENT-16, a randomized, double-blind, placebo-controlled trial evaluating the addition of sintilimab, a monoclonal antibody to PD-1, to first-line chemotherapy in patients with advanced esophagogastric adenocarcinoma. Patients received capecitabine and oxaliplatin every 3 weeks combined with either placebo or sintilimab (3 mg/kg in patients <60 kg or 200 mg in patients >60 kg) for up to six cycles.

Of the 650 patients enrolled, 81% had gastric primary tumors, 39% had liver metastases, and 61% had PD-L1 combined positive scores (CPS) >5%. The primary endpoint of overall survival was improved with sintilimab compared with placebo in patients with CPS >5% (median, 18.4 vs. 12.9 months; hazard ratio, 0.66; *p*=0.002) and in all randomized patients (median,15.2 vs. 12.3 months; HR, 0.77; *p*=0.009).

No survival benefit with sintilimab was seen in patients with CPS <5% (HR, 0.90). Among patients with CPS >5% PFS was improved with sintilimab over placebo (7.7 vs. 5.8 months; HR, 0.63; *p*< 0.001) as was response rate (63.6% vs. 49.4%, respectively; *p*=0.008).

This trial adds sintilimab to the list of anti–PD-1 agents that improve outcomes when added to first-line chemotherapy in metastatic esophagogastric adenocarcinoma. As with the other positive trials, survival improvements were limited to patients with PDL-1 CPS >5%.

- **The Best Treatment Approach for Locally Advanced Esophageal Cancer[99]**

*The findings favored preoperative triplet chemotherapy (adding docetaxel to cisplatin/5-FU) over doublet chemotherapy. Adding radiotherapy to doublet chemotherapy was not superior to doublet or triplet chemotherapy alone. For patients with non-operative esophageal squamous cancers, chemoradiotherapy remains the standard of care.*

Japanese investigators compared three neoadjuvant treatments in 601 patients with locally advanced esophageal squamous cancer in an open-label, randomized, multicenter trial.

The three protocols were:

1. 5-day infusion of 5-FU with 1 day of cisplatin for two 3-week cycles
2. The same regimen plus 1 day of docetaxel, for three 3-week cycles
3. 4-day infusion of 5-FU and 1 day of cisplatin for two 4-week cycles plus concurrent radiotherapy (total dose, 41.4 Gy)

At a median follow-up of 50.7 months, the primary endpoint of 3-year overall survival (OS) was significantly superior with docetaxel triplet chemotherapy compared to doublet chemotherapy (72.1% vs. 62.6%); triplet chemotherapy also showed superior 3-year progression-free survival. Pathologic complete response was also higher with triplet than doublet chemotherapy (19.8% vs. 2.0%).

- **Does Sorafenib Add Benefit to TACE in HCC?[92]**

*The addition of the tyrosine kinase inhibitor sorafenib significantly improved overall and progression-free survival compared with transarterial chemoembolization (TACE) alone in patients with recurrent intermediate-stage hepatocellular cancer.*

In this multicenter, open-label, randomized, phase 3 trial comparing TACE alone or combined with sorafenib (400 mg twice daily; SOR-TACE) in 162 patients in China with recurrent intermediate-stage HCC. In this trial HCC was defined as multifocal disease confined to the liver without vascular invasion or extrahepatic spread, who had positive microvascular invasion after prior potentially curative surgery. Most patients had hepatitis B (91%) and cirrhosis (62%), and most had more than 3 tumors (92%) with a median size less than 5 cm (81%); 33% underwent one TACE session, 27% underwent two, and 40% underwent three or more sessions.

At a median follow-up of 37.5 months, the primary endpoint of overall survival was superior for SOR-TACE compared to TACE (median, 22.2 vs. 15.1 months, $p<0.01$), with superior survival at 12 months (90.1% vs. 71.6%), 24 months (44.4% vs. 24.2%), and 36 months (26.9% vs. 13.6%). Progression-free survival was also superior for SOR-TACE over TACE (median, 16.2 vs. 11.8 months, p<001).

These findings show that adding a systemic agent to regional therapy improves survival in patients with HCC. It is likely that this approach will be used with the superior first-line immunotherapies that are now available.

## CHAPTER 16. BILIARY TRACT CANCER

- **Trastuzumab Deruxtecan for HER2-Positive Biliary Cancer?**[96]

*More than one third of patients with HER2+ biliary cancer had a response to the antibody–drug conjugate trastuzumab deruxtecan (T-DXd) in a small, single-arm study from Japan. T-DXd was granted accelerated approval by the USA FDA for use in patients with any advanced HER2+ solid tumors. Given the potential for use of targeted therapy in advanced biliary cancer, testing for biomarkers such as HER2 and performing next generation sequencing should now be performed in these patients*

Biliary cancers frequently harbor targetable mutations and gene amplified pathways, including IDH-1, FGFR2, BRAF V600E, and human epidermal growth factor receptor 2 (HER2). There is increasing evidence that a range of HER2-targeted therapies are active in HER2-positive biliary cancer.

Investigators in Japan reported the results of a single-arm, phase 2 trial of the antibody–drug conjugate trastuzumab deruxtecan (T-DXd) in HER2-expressing advanced biliary cancer. Central pathologic confirmation of HER2 status by both immunohistochemistry and in situ hybridization was performed in archival tissue from 296 patients, of whom 61 (20.6%) tested HER2+. Thirty eligible patients were treated with T-DXd (5.4 mg/kg every 3 weeks), including 22 with HER2+ and 8 with HER2 low disease. Most patients had primary gallbladder tumors (43.3%), followed by extrahepatic (26.7%) and intrahepatic (20.0%) biliary cancers.

The response rate in the 22 HER2+ patients was 36.4%. One of eight patients (12.5%) with HER2-low disease had a response. The median duration of response in the HER2+ patients was 7.4 months, and the median overall survival was 7.1 months. Two patients (6.0%) had fatal treatment-related interstitial lung disease.

Careful monitoring for pulmonary toxicity to avoid potentially fatal drug-related interstitial lung disease is required.

- **A promising first-line treatment for neuroendocrine tumors (NETs)[6]**

*Progression-free survival was superior with $^{177}$Lu-Dotatate plus octreotide LAR compared with octreotide LAR alone.*

Investigators reported results of the NETTER-2 trial evaluating first-line therapy in somatostatin receptor–positive grade 2 and 3 well-differentiated gastroenteropancreatic (GEP) NETs. In this open-label, phase 3 trial, patients were randomized to treatment with $^{177}$Lu-Dotatate combined with octreotide long-acting repeatable (LAR; 30 mg every 8 weeks) or octreotide LAR alone (60 mg every 4 weeks). Of the 226 patients, 54% had pancreatic and 29% had small-intestinal primary tumors; 65% had grade 2 and 35% had grade 3 NETS; 90% had hepatic and 60% had lymph node metastases.

The primary endpoint of progression-free survival was superior with $^{177}$Lu-Dotatate plus octreotide LAR compared with octreotide LAR alone (median, 22.8 vs. 8.5 months; hazard ratio, 0.276; $p<0.0001$). Response rate also was superior with $^{177}$Lu-Dotatate plus octreotide LAR over octreotide LAR alone (43% vs. 9.3%; odds ratio, 7.81; $p<0.0001$). Time to deterioration in quality of life did not differ between groups. Overall survival results are pending.

One case of myelodysplastic syndrome occurred in the $^{177}$Lu-Dotatate arm, but no new adverse events were observed.

**A Phase 3 Trial of Cabozantinib to Treat Advanced Neuroendocrine Tumors[79]**

*Progression-free survival with cabozantinib was better compared to placebo*

The investigators performed a phase 3 trial of cabozantinib in patients who either extrapancreatic neuroendocrine tumors or who had pancreatic neuroendocrine tumors, and who had received peptide receptor radionuclide therapy or targeted therapy or both. Cabozantinib is an oral small-molecule inhibitor of multiple tyrosine kinases including VEGF receptors, MET, AXL, and RET.

In the cohort of 203 patients with extrapancreatic neuroendocrine tumors, the median progression-free survival with cabozantinib was 8.4 months, compared with 3.9 months with placebo ($p<0.001$).

In the cohort of 95 patients with pancreatic neuroendocrine tumors, the median progression-free survival with cabozantinib was 13.8 months, compared with 4.4 months with placebo ($p<0.001$). The incidence of confirmed objective response with cabozantinib was 5% and 19% among patients with extrapancreatic and pancreatic neuroendocrine tumors,

- **Brigatinib in NF2-Related Schwannomatosis with Progressive Tumors[76]**

*Brigatinib treatment resulted in radiographic responses in multiple tumor types and clinical benefit*

NF2-related schwannomatosis (NF2-SWN), formerly called neurofibromatosis type 2) is a tumor predisposition syndrome that is manifested by multiple vestibular schwannomas, nonvestibular schwannomas, meningiomas, and ependymomas. The condition is relentlessly progressive with no approved therapies. Surgery remains the standard of care, but the risk of iatrogenic neurologic injury increases with each surgery. Chemotherapy offers the possibility of treating multiple tumors without the risk of surgical complications. The majority of completed trials have studied a single drug targeting a single tumor type (vestibular schwannoma). On the basis of preclinical activity of brigatinib (an inhibitor of multiple tyrosine kinases) in NF2-driven nonvestibular schwannoma and meningioma, data were needed on the use of brigatinib in patients with multiple types of progressive NF2-SWN tumors.

In this phase 2 platform trial with a basket design, patients who were 12 years of age or older with NF2-SWN and progressive tumors were treated with oral brigatinib at a dose of 180 mg daily. The primary outcome was radiographic response in target tumors. Key secondary outcomes were safety, response rate in all tumors, hearing response, and patient-reported outcomes.

A total of 40 patients (median age, 26 years) with progressive target tumors (10 vestibular schwannomas, 8 nonvestibular schwannomas, 20 meningiomas, and 2 ependymomas) received treatment with brigatinib. After a median follow-up of 10.4

months, the percentage of tumors with a radiographic response was 10% for target tumors and 23% for all tumors; meningiomas and nonvestibular schwannomas had the greatest benefit. Annualized growth rates decreased for all tumor types during treatment. Hearing improvement occurred in 35% of eligible ears. Exploratory analyses suggested a decrease in self-reported pain severity during treatment. No grade 4 or 5 treatment-related adverse events were reported.

Brigatinib treatment resulted in radiographic responses in multiple tumor types and clinical benefit in a heavily pretreated cohort of patients with NF2-SWN.

## CHAPTER 18. CANCER OF UNKNOWN PRIMARY

- **Molecularly Targeted Treatment for Cancer of Unknown Primary (CUP)[98]**

*The standard of care for CUP usually involves generic chemotherapy regimens with poor outcomes. This study's approach holds the promise that more-nuanced therapy recommendations based on molecular profiling could improve outcomes and might be further enhanced when more targeted agents become available.*

Cancer of unknown primary (CUP) has been associated with a poor prognosis, short survival, and treatment approaches that typically utilize generic chemotherapy regimens with antitumor activity in the most likely primary sites of disease. These regimens often are platinum- or taxane-based combinations and are associated with little improvement in overall survival (OS).

To determine the effect of a molecularly guided treatment (MGT) of CUP, the investigators conducted a multinational, phase 2, open-label trial. They enrolled 636 patients with non-squamous CUP and good functional status who were eligible for platinum-based chemotherapy and had tumor tissue or liquid biopsy material available for gene expression profiling. Patients first received three cycles of induction chemotherapy with a platinum-based regimen (carboplatin-paclitaxel, cisplatin-gemcitabine, or carboplatin-gemcitabine). Those with tumor response or stable disease (n=436) were then randomized to either MGT or continuation of the same chemotherapy. Patients randomized to the MGT group who did not have a targetable alteration, high tumor mutational burden, or high microsatellite instability were treated with chemotherapy plus the immune checkpoint inhibitor atezolizumab, which targets the programmed death ligand 1 (PD-L1)

Median follow-up was 24 months. Median progression-free survival (PFS) was 6.1 months in the MGT group and 4.4 months in the chemotherapy group (p=0.0079).

## Chapter 19. CHRONIC MYELOID LEUKEMIA (CML)

- **Front-line asciminib for chronic myeloid leukemia**[3,88]

*In this trial comparing asciminib with investigator-selected TKIs and imatinib, asciminib showed superior efficacy and a favorable safety profile in patients with newly diagnosed chronic-phase CML.*

First- and second-generation tyrosine kinase inhibitors (TKIs) targeting the BCR/ABL1 chimeric protein offer durable remission for many patients with chronic myeloid leukemia (CML), but resistance develops in the setting of ATP active-site mutations. Asciminib, a TKI that binds to the ABL myristoyl pocket, is approved for patients with CML who have failed to respond to two prior TKIs due to resistance or treatment intolerance. Investigators reported on a randomized, phase 3 trial comparing asciminib (80 mg once daily) with investigator's choice of imatinib or a second-generation TKI (nilotinib, dasatinib, or bosutinib) in 405 adults with newly diagnosed chronic-phase CML. They found that asciminib improved responses and lowered toxicity compared to traditional, previously used tyrosine kinase inhibitors for CML.

## Chapter 20. CHRONIC LYMPHOCYTIC LEUKEMIA (CLL)

- **MRD-Guided Ibrutinib plus Venetoclax in Untreated CLL**[66]

*The combination provided superior progression-free survival compared to fludarabine, cyclophosphamide, and rituximab.*

Targeted therapeutics - Bruton tyrosine kinase inhibitors (BTKi), anti-CD20 monoclonal antibodies, and the BCL2 inhibitor venetoclax - have become the mainstays of treatment for chronic lymphocytic leukemia (CLL). To investigate the combination of the BTKi ibrutinib plus venetoclax (Ibr/Ven) versus fludarabine, cyclophosphamide, and rituximab (FCR), investigators in the U.K. conducted a multicenter, open-label, phase 3 trial in 523 patients with previously untreated CLL.

In the Ibr/Ven group, the duration of treatment was determined by measurable residual disease (MRD) assessed by multiparameter flow cytometry in peripheral blood and bone marrow. Patients with >20% del(17p) were excluded from the study.

At a median follow-up of 44 months, disease progression or death had occurred in 12 patients in the Ibr/Ven group versus 75 in the FCR group (hazard ratio, 0.13). Estimated 3-year progression-free survival was 97% vs. 77%, respectively. Overall survival favored Ibr/Ven, with an estimated rate at 3 years of 98% versus 93% with FCR. At 3 years, 58% of patients in the Ibr/Ven group had stopped treatment because they achieved undetectable MRD (sensitivity threshold, 1 in $10^4$ cells). Serious blood and lymphatic events occurred in 5% of the Ibr/Ven group versus 31% of the FCR group, whereas serious cardiac events occurred in 10.7% versus 0.4%. Secondary cancers including myeloid malignancies were more frequent in the FCR group.

Longer follow-up of the FLAIR trial confirms the high efficacy of Ibr/Ven compared to the historical standard regime, FCR, with particular benefit from Ibr/Ven in the cohort with *IGHV*-unmutated CLL. MRD-guided therapy allowed patients in the Ibr/Ven group to discontinue treatment at 3- and 5-year timepoints. The severe cardiac adverse events in the Ibr/Ven arm indicate the need for careful patient selection for ibrutinib therapy in the setting of pre-existing cardiac disease.

## Chapter 21. ACUTE MYELOID LEUKEMIA AND ACUTE LYMPHOBLASTIC LEUKEMIA

- **CAR T Cell Therapy for Relapsed Acute Myeloid and Acute Lymphoblastic Leukemia[20,21]**

*In a pilot study, sequential anti-CD7 CAR T-cell infusion followed by haploidentical allogeneic hematopoietic stem-cell transplantation produced ongoing remission.*

While chimeric antigen receptor (CAR) T-cell therapies are now a standard treatment for relapsed or refractory B-cell malignancies, their application in myeloid and T-cell neoplasms has lagged behind, in part due to effects on normal hematopoiesis. Investigators recently reported a novel approach of induction therapy with an anti-CD7 CAR T-cell product followed by hematopoietic reconstitution using haploidentical allogeneic hematopoietic stem-cell transplantation (alloHSCT).

Seventeen patients with relapsed CD7-positive acute myeloid leukemia (AML) or T-cell acute lymphoblastic leukemia (ALL)/lymphoblastic lymphoma received a haploidentical donor-derived anti-CD7 CAR-T infusion. Of those, 10 patients achieved complete remission with incomplete hematologic recovery and severe marrow hypocellularity, plus detectable circulating CD7 CAR T cells, and were eligible for haploidentical alloHSCT using the original T-cell donor. Conditioning chemotherapy (fludarabine, cyclophosphamide, and etoposide) was given prior to CAR T-cell infusion. No further conditioning was given prior to the administration of the allo-HSCT. Furthermore, no pre- or post-alloHSCT graft-versus-host disease (GVHD) prophylaxis was administered.

One patient died of infection 13 days after HSCT, eight had successful engraftment, and one had autologous blood count recovery. Another patient later died from infection, and two from CD7-negative leukemia relapse. At a median follow-up of 15.1 months, six patients remained in ongoing remission. Estimated 1-year disease-free survival was 54%. No cytokine release syndrome occurred; grade 1–2 acute GVHD was observed in three patients, with no chronic GVHD.

This complex trial provides proof of principle demonstrating the efficacy of coupled anti-CD7 CAR T-cell therapy and alloHSCT in patients with relapsed, poor-risk AML and T-cell ALL. The haplo-donor strategy illustrates a pathway for CAR T-cell therapy in neoplasms where obtaining donor T cells is not feasible. Further study is warranted with CD7 and other leukemic cell targets.

## CHAPTER 22. ACUTE LYMPHOBLASTIC LEUKEMIA (ALL)

- **Blinatumomab for MRD-Negative Acute Lymphoblastic Leukemia in Adults[4]**

*The addition of blinatumomab to consolidation chemotherapy has significantly improved survival in patients with Philadelphia chromosome-negative pre-B-cell acute lymphoblastic leukemia.*

To evaluate a strategy to further improve outcomes, investigators conducted a multicenter, randomized, phase 3 trial comparing the anti-CD19/anti-CD3 T-cell–engaging bispecific antibody blinatumomab in combination with four cycles of consolidation chemotherapy versus chemotherapy alone. At a median follow-up of 43 months, a planned interim analysis showed the 3-year overall survival OS) to be 85% in the blinatumomab arm versus 68% with chemotherapy alone (hazard ratio, 0.41; $p<0.002$). Three-year relapse-free survival was also significantly improved with blinatumomab (80% vs. 68%). This is a practice-changing report and further studies are warranted.

- **Remission from B-Cell ALL with Chemotherapy-Free Induction Therapy[49]**

*Durable remission was achieved with front-line dasatinib plus blinatumomab in adults with Philadelphia chromosome-positive acute lymphoblastic leukemia.*

Tyrosine kinase inhibitors (TKIs) targeting BCR-ABL are an integral component of initial therapy for Philadelphia chromosome-positive acute lymphoblastic leukemia (Ph+ ALL). Investigators from the multicenter, phase 2 D-ALBA trial reported long-term outcomes for 63 patients (age range, 24–82; median, 54) treated with the TKI dasatinib plus the CD19/CD3 T-cell–engaging bispecific monoclonal antibody blinatumomab. Patients received 12-week cycles of corticosteroids for 7 days, dasatinib (140 mg/day) plus corticosteroids for 23 days, and dasatinib alone for 54 days. Daily dasatinib was continued during consolidation with 2 or more cycles of blinatumomab. Central nervous system prophylaxis was administered via lumbar puncture at multiple time points. Serial minimal residual disease was analyzed in bone marrow by reverse transcriptase-polymerase chain reaction.

The complete remission rate was 98%. The molecular response rate was 60% following cycle 2 of blinatumomab and increased to 93% at 12 months. At a median follow-up of 53 months, disease-free survival (DFS) was 75.8%, and overall survival was 80.7%. DFS was significantly lower in patients without molecular response at the end of induction and in those with the $IKZF_1^{plus}$ mutation. Of 29 patients treated with ongoing TKI therapy but not cytotoxic chemotherapy or stem cell transplantation, 28 remained in complete hematologic remission at a median 48 months of follow-up.

These long-term results of the D-ALBA trial confirm the efficacy of chemotherapy-free induction and maintenance therapy in adults with Ph+ ALL. The DFS was 100% for patients in molecular remission at the end of induction, which confirms the prognostic benefit of this metric. The combination of ponatinib plus blinatumomab has shown similar promising results, and additional multicenter chemotherapy-free and risk-adapted trials are in progress.

- **Effective De-Escalation of B-Cell ALL Induction Therapy[59,60]**

*Complete remission was achieved with inotuzumab ozogamicin plus dexamethasone induction therapy in older adults with Philadelphia chromosome–negative precursor B-cell ALL.*

The anti-CD22 antibody-drug conjugate inotuzumab ozogamicin (InO) provides high response rates in relapsed or refractory B-cell acute lymphoblastic leukemia (ALL). To explore its efficacy and safety in the frontline setting, investigators in Germany conducted a prospective, multicenter, phase 2 trial in 45 patients older than 55 years with newly diagnosed Philadelphia chromosome–negative, CD22-expressing precursor-B-cell ALL.

Induction therapy included 2 or 3 cycles of InO plus dexamethasone, followed by age-adapted consolidation (5 cycles), late intensification (1 cycle), and maintenance chemotherapy (up to 2 years). Intrathecal chemotherapy prophylaxis was administered during all treatment phases. Serial measurable residual disease (MRD) testing was performed by flow cytometry (minimum sensitivity, 1 in $10^4$ cells).

The 43 evaluable patients had a median age of 64 (range, 56–80); 3 had central nervous system involvement at diagnosis, and 12 had high-risk cytogenetic alterations. All patients achieved complete remission (CR) or CR with incomplete peripheral blood count recovery; 53% were MRD negative after two InO cycles, 71% after 3 cycles. With a median follow-up of 2.7 years, 1-year event-free survival (EFS; the primary study endpoint) was 88% and 3-year EFS was 55%. Toxicities during InO cycles occurred mostly in cycle 1 and included cytopenias (58%–74%; most grade 3–4), elevated bilirubin (21%, grade 3–4 in 2%), and elevated transaminases (37%, grade 3–4 in 14%). One patient developed hepatic veno-occlusive disease during cycle 2 of InO induction.

Older adults with Philadelphia chromosome-negative B-ALL have poor outcomes with traditional multiagent chemotherapy regimens due to leukemia resistance and treatment-related toxicities. InO plus dexamethasone induction was highly efficacious and well-tolerated in this study with most patients achieving MRD-negative complete remission, and further exploration in prospective randomized trials is warranted.

- **ViPOR: A New Regimen for Treating Aggressive Lymphoma?[7]**

*Combining five therapeutic agents led to durable remission in a subset of patients with relapsed B-cell lymphoma.*

Researchers investigated whether targeting multiple cellular pathways with a combination of medications might improve remission rates.

Patients with relapsed/refractory (R/R) diffuse large B-cell lymphoma (DLBCL) received the oral agents venetoclax (a B-cell lymphoma 2 inhibitor), ibrutinib (a Bruton tyrosine kinase inhibitor), prednisone, and lenalidomide (an immunomodulatory agent) plus the anti-CD20 monoclonal antibody obinutuzumab. The regimen, referred to as ViPOR, was administered every 21 days for six cycles, with the oral drugs administered on days 1 through 14 (prednisone for 7 days) and obinutuzumab given intravenously on days 1 and 2.

Among the 48 patients with evaluable data, the proportion with a complete response (CR) differed by DLBCL subtype: germinal center B-cell (GCB), 0/12; non-GCB, 8/13 (62%); double-hit *MYC/BCL2*, 8/15 (53%); and other, 2/8 (25%). A 2-year duration of response was seen in 65% of all responding patients and 78% of those who achieved CR.

- **Replacing Autologous Stem Cell Transplantation in Mantle Cell Lymphoma?[17,18]**

*Adding ibrutinib to induction and maintenance therapy improved outcomes, including patients with poor-risk disease.*

Prior phase 3 trials established autologous stem cell transplant (ASCT) consolidation and maintenance rituximab as standards of care in younger, transplant-eligible patients with previously untreated mantle cell lymphoma (MCL). Now, investigators report a multinational, phase 3 trial testing incorporation of the Bruton tyrosine kinase inhibitor (BTKi) ibrutinib into induction and maintenance therapy.

A total of 870 patients (median age, 57 years; 76% male; 98% white) were randomized to one of three regimens:

a). Six alternating cycles of rituximab, cyclophosphamide, doxorubicin, vincristine, and prednisone (R-CHOP) and rituximab, dexamethasone, cytarabine, and cisplatin (R-DHAP), followed by ASCT consolidation in responding patients (arm A)

b). The above regimen plus ibrutinib added to R-CHOP cycles and 2 years of ibrutinib maintenance therapy, with ASCT for responding patients (arm A+I)

c). The A+I regimen without ASCT (arm I)

Patients in each arm also could receive rituximab maintenance according to local guidelines.

At a median follow-up of 31 months, 3-year failure-free survival (FFS; the primary outcome) was superior for arm A+I compared with arm A (88% vs. 72%; hazard ratio, 0.52; *p*=0.0008). FFS favored arm I over arm A (86% vs. 72%) but the difference did not reach statistical significance (HR, 1.77). Outcomes for patients with poor-risk mantle cell lymphoma international prognostic index (MIPI) scores and p53 overexpression were significantly improved in the ibrutinib-containing arms compared with arm A. Grade 3–5 toxicities were similar during induction therapy with and without ibrutinib; however, adverse hematologic and infectious events were higher during maintenance therapy in arm A+I.

This practice-changing study demonstrates a clear benefit for incorporating ibrutinib into induction and maintenance therapy, although the data as yet are inconclusive regarding elimination of high-dose chemotherapy plus ASCT. This trial shows a pathway toward de-escalated treatment intensity and improved outcomes in younger patients with MCL.

- **CAR T-Cell Therapy for Mantle-Cell Lymphoma[22]**

*Lisocabtagene maraleucel produced high remission rates in patients with relapsed or refractory disease, with encouraging activity in CNS lymphoma and low rates of grade 3 or 4 toxicities.*

Chimeric antigen receptor (CAR) T-cell immunotherapy provides an important option for relapsed or refractory mantle-cell lymphoma (MCL). Investigators now report a multicenter, phase 1 study of lisocabtagene maraleucel (liso-cel) in patients whose

MCL had progressed after two or more lines of therapy, including an anti-CD20 agent, an alkylator, and a Bruton tyrosine kinase inhibitor. Bridging therapy was permitted after leukapheresis; patients received lymphodepleting fludarabine plus cyclophosphamide for 3 days and then liso-cel infusions 2 to 7 days later (total dose, 50 or 100 x $10^6$ cells). Retreatment with liso-cel was permitted for patients who relapsed after complete remission.

Of the 104 patients who underwent leukapheresis, 88 received liso-cel (82 at the 100 x $10^6$ dose); 9 patients died before infusion, 3 did not meet eligibility criteria, and 4 received a nonconforming CAR T-cell product. Among 83 evaluable patients, the overall response rate was 83.1%, with complete remission achieved in 72.3%, including 11 of 19 with *TP53* mutations, 17 of 27 with blastoid variant, and 6 of 7 with central nervous system (CNS) MCL. During a median follow-up of 23.5 months, the median progression-free survival was 15.3 months and overall survival was 18.2 months. Cytokine release syndrome occurred in 61% of patients (all grade 1 or 2 apart from one grade 4 event) and neurotoxicity in 31%, with seven (8%) grade-3 events and one (1%) grade 4. There were three treatment-related deaths, two from infections and one from tumor lysis syndrome. Seven patients died of COVID-19.

Liso-cel produced high response rates and durable remission in patients with multi-resistant, heavily pretreated MCL, including those with high-risk features, CNS MCL, and age ≥65. Toxicities appear to compare favorably with other CAR T-cell therapies and bispecific monoclonal antibodies. Longer follow-up is needed for durability of response, including the cohort of patients receiving a second liso-cel infusion. Analysis of liso-cel earlier in therapy is warranted.

- **Bispecific Immunotherapy for Relapsed/Refractory Lymphoma[26]**

*Durable remission was achieved in indolent and aggressive subtypes of B-cell lymphomas with the bispecific monoclonal antibody mosunetuzumab.*

Bispecific T-cell engaging monoclonal antibodies have emerged as important options for patients with relapsed or refractory (R/R) B-cell malignancies. Investigators now report extended follow-up from a multicenter, phase 1/2 trial of mosunetuzumab, a

CD20 x CD3 bispecific antibody, in patients with R/R indolent and aggressive B-cell non-Hodgkin lymphoma (iNHL and aNHL).

Mosunetuzumab was administered intravenously in 21-day cycles using a stepped-up dosing schedule in cycle 1, with corticosteroid premedication to mitigate infusion reactions and cytokine release syndrome during the first 2 cycles (optional with subsequent cycles); a dose of 30 mg on day 1 was administered beginning with cycle 3. Patients achieving complete response (CR) could discontinue treatment.

A total of 196 patients were treated with the full-dose regimen. At a median follow-up of 3.5 years (range 2.7–6.3 years), the overall (partial and complete) response rates were 65.7% (44/67) in patients with iNHL and 36.4% (47/129) in those with aNHL. Among patients with iNHL who achieved CR, no relapses were observed after 26 months. Among all patients with iNHL, 36-month progression-free survival (PFS) was 29.7%. In patients with aNHL, the median duration of response was 7.8 months (28.8 months for those with CR) and 36-month PFS was 10.3%. Of 12 patients with CR (8 iNHL; 4 aNHL) who were retreated with mosunetuzumab after prior discontinuation of therapy, 10 responded, including 7 who had a second CR. No new adverse events were observed.

Bispecific antibodies have joined the anti-CD20 monoclonal antibodies, antibody–drug conjugates, and CAR-T immunotherapeutic armamentarium for B-cell lymphomas. This longer-term follow-up of the pivotal mosunetuzumab trial further supports its use in relapsed iNHL and aNHL. Mosunetuzumab offers benefits of time-limited therapy for complete responders, off-the-shelf availability (unlike CAR-T cells), and response with retreatment. Ongoing studies are addressing its use in earlier in therapy.

- **High-Dose Chemotherapy for Primary Central Nervous System Lymphoma[38]**

*Almost 60% of patients older than 65 achieved a 12-month progression-free survival after intensive induction therapy and consolidative autologous stem-cell transplantation.*

Outcomes for primary central nervous system lymphoma (PCNSL) have been improved via intensive immunochemotherapy plus autologous stem-cell transplantation (ASCT) consolidation, although clinicians have been concerned that older patients cannot benefit from this regimen due to underlying comorbidities and treatment-related toxicities. In MARTA, a phase 2, prospective, single-arm, German multicenter trial, researchers investigated the use of CNS-penetrating high-dose therapy and ASCT consolidation in 54 fit patients 65 years or older with newly diagnosed PCNSL. Eligible patients received two cycles of high-dose methotrexate and cytarabine plus rituximab, followed by a conditioning regimen of rituximab, thiotepa, and busulfan and then ASCT rescue.

In the 51 evaluable patients, the 12-month progression-free survival (the primary endpoint) was 58.8%, but this did not meet the statistical threshold for efficacy. The 1-year overall survival was 80.6% among the 36 patients completing study treatment. At a median follow-up of 23 months, 23 patients (45%) had progression or relapse of disease or had died. Seven deaths occurred during induction and consolidation; three were considered treatment-related.

These findings from MARTA suggest that carefully selected, older PCNSL patients treated at specialized centers can benefit from high-dose chemotherapy and ASCT. The considerable need for effective treatment remains unmet among both younger and older patients with significant comorbidities and among those whose disease relapses or is refractory to initial therapy. Promising early data have led to an ongoing clinical trial exploring the integration of targeted agents plus immunochemotherapy (TEDDI-R regimen).

- **T-Cell Immunotherapy for Posttransplant EBV-Positive Lymphoma[39]**

*Half of patients with relapsed/refractory EBV-positive posttransplant lymphoproliferative disorder responded to tabelecleucel, an allogeneic T-cell immunotherapeutic agent.*

Epstein–Barr virus (EBV)–positive posttransplant lymphoproliferative disorder (PTLD) is a well-recognized complication of hematopoietic stem cell transplantation

(HSCT) and solid organ transplantation (SOT). Patients who do not respond to a decrease in immunosuppressive therapy, rituximab, or rituximab plus chemotherapy have a very poor prognosis. Investigators now report updated safety and efficacy findings from a phase 3, single-arm, open-label, multicenter trial of tabelecleucel, an allogeneic EBV-specific T-cell immunotherapeutic agent, in patients with relapsed or refractory EBV-positive PTLD.

A dose of $2 \times 10^6$ cells/kg was administered intravenously on days 1, 8, and 15 in 35-day cycles, followed by observation. Any non-responders could be retreated with tabelecleucel using a T-cell line with a different human leukocyte antigen (HLA) restriction. Treatment ended with achievement of maximal response, intolerable toxicity, start of non-protocol therapy, or failure of tabelecleucel with up to four (for HSCT) or two (for SOT) different HLA restrictions.

Of 63 patients assessed for eligibility for participation, 43 were included in the trial. Among these 43 patients, an objective response (primary endpoint) was achieved in 7/14 (50%) in the HSCT patient group, with a median follow-up of 14.1 months, and in 15/29 (52%) in the SOT group, with a median follow-up of 6 months. Nine patients progressed on treatment. There was no evidence of cytokine release syndrome, tumor flare, or neurotoxicity syndrome as is seen with autologous chimeric antigen receptor (CAR) T-cell agents; no fatal treatment-related adverse events were reported. One patient developed grade 1 chronic graft-versus-host disease.

This allogeneic T-cell immunotherapy showed promising activity and safety in a rare but challenging posttransplant, high-grade lymphoma. Other off-the-shelf cell therapeutics also are in development for a spectrum of hematologic malignancies that may expand patient eligibility and more-rapid access to CAR-T therapy.

- **Minimal Residual Disease Predicts Outcome in Follicular Lymphoma[46]**

*Achieving undetectable MRD significantly increased progression-free and overall survival, especially for patients with an early MRD response to induction therapy.*

Achievement of minimal residual disease (MRD) negativity in peripheral blood and bone marrow correlates with improved outcomes in patients with B cell non-Hodgkin lymphoma. Investigators evaluated the prognostic value of MRD status in patients with advanced follicular lymphoma undergoing immunochemotherapy in a multicenter, phase 3 trial (GALLIUM).

Previously untreated patients were randomized to induction with rituximab or obinutuzumab plus chemotherapy, followed by maintenance with the assigned antibody for 2 years. MRD was assessed by nested and quantitative polymerase chain reaction (PCR) for clonal immunoglobulin gene rearrangement and the t(14;18) breakpoint; positive MRD was indicated if both assays were detectable at or above 1 in$10^4$ sensitivity. Samples were collected from blood, bone marrow, or both during and at the end of induction and maintenance therapy.

Of 1064 enrolled patients, 249 (23.4%) had no clonal PCR marker detected or had samples that did not meet MRD evaluability metrics. At a median follow-up of 59 months, MRD positivity at the middle or end of induction was significantly associated with poorer progression-free survival (PFS) and overall survival (OS) and a higher rate of disease progression within 24 months compared with MRD negativity. Three-year PFS was 81.1% for patients who were positron emission tomography (PET)-negative/MRD-negative at the end of induction, versus 58.8% of those PET-negative/MRD-positive and 73.9% of those PET-positive/MRD-negative. Persistent or recurrent MRD-positivity during maintenance therapy correlated strongly with clinical relapse and poorer outcome. MRD-negativity rates were higher in patients treated with bendamustine versus other chemotherapies and in those treated with obinutuzumab versus rituximab.

MRD status assessed with PCR-based assays provided a robust biomarker for outcomes in patients with advanced follicular lymphoma treated with immunochemotherapy. However, MRD status predicted only 25% of the poor-risk subgroup that progressed within 24 months of treatment. Use of current next-generation sequencing methodologies will be of interest given their greater sensitivity and detection of an informative marker for more patients. MRD warrants further analysis in prospective, risk-adapted follicular lymphoma clinical trials.

- **Postinduction Maintenance Therapy in Mantle Cell Lymphoma**[63]

*Patients with MCL who achieve undetectable minimal residual disease status after induction therapy benefit significantly from maintenance rituximab; as such, maintenance rituximab should not be withheld in this setting.*

Achievement of complete remission and undetectable minimal residual disease (MRD) status following induction immunochemotherapy is associated with improved outcomes for patients with mantle cell lymphoma (MCL). Investigators now report long-term follow-up of the European MCL Elderly Trial in which 560 patients ≥60 years of age, who were not eligible for autologous stem cell transplant consolidation, were randomized to either R-CHOP (rituximab, cyclophosphamide, doxorubicin, vincristine, prednisone) for 8 cycles or R-FC (rituximab, fludarabine, cyclophosphamide) for 6 cycles; patients with complete or partial remission were then randomized to either maintenance rituximab or interferon-alpha.

Serial MRD determinations were made using real-time quantitative PCR (median sensitivity, $1 \times 10^{-5}$) on peripheral blood and bone marrow samples during induction and maintenance therapy. The aims of this long-term follow-up were to determine if end-of-induction MRD status influenced the benefit of rituximab maintenance and whether de-escalation of maintenance therapy should be encouraged in MRD-negative patients.

Greater rates of MRD negativity were achieved with R-FC but with poorer overall survival (OS) versus R-CHOP, in part due to toxicity. Maintenance rituximab significantly improved outcomes compared with interferon. Informative end-of-induction MRD samples were available for 171 of 217 (79%) patients treated in France or Germany who had not progressed during induction therapy. In the R-CHOP arm, both progression-free survival and OS were significantly improved (hazard ratios, 0.23 and 0.19, respectively) in those who were MRD negative at the end of induction and who received maintenance rituximab. MRD-positive patients had less benefit from maintenance rituximab and an earlier time to progression.

This analysis confirmed the significant benefit of maintenance rituximab following R-CHOP induction in patients who are MRD negative at the end of induction, thus refuting an approach that would de-escalate use of maintenance therapy in this setting. Alternative consolidation or maintenance therapies need to be explored for patients who are MRD positive after induction, given their short time to progression despite maintenance rituximab.

## Chapter 24. MYELOMA AND MONOCLONAL GAMMOPATHY

- **A Model for Managing Patients with Monoclonal Gammopathy of Undetermined Significance[37]**

*A new prediction model indicates which patients with MGUS should be considered for bone marrow sampling.*

About 1,000 people (median age, 68) with presumed MGUS underwent bone marrow sampling; those with the IgM isotype were excluded. The researchers developed a multivariable model to predict ≥10% plasma cells - indicating a diagnosis of smouldering multiple myeloma - on bone marrow examination. The model incorporated MGUS isotype (i.e., IgG, IgA, light chain, or biclonal), monoclonal protein concentration, free light chain ratio, and total concentrations of IgG, IgA, and IgM.

The model's performance for predicting ≥10% plasma cells in bone marrow was as follows:

Sensitivity was 86% (14% of cases were missed).

Specificity was 67% (33% of patients with <10% plasma cells were incorrectly predicted to have ≥10%).

Specificity was substantially better than that of the Mayo Clinic model, applied to this cohort (67% vs. 41%); sensitivities were similar in the two models.

Assuming a goal of identifying patients with ≥10% plasma cells, this model would have allowed deferral of bone marrow sampling in 59% of patients in this cohort (compared with 37% using the Mayo Clinic model).

For primary care clinicians who diagnose MGUS (which requires absence of symptoms or signs of myeloma or related conditions), this model could inform decisions on whether to refer patients for possible bone marrow sampling.

**Daratumumab for Newly Diagnosed Multiple Myeloma[68]**

*In transplant-eligible patients, the addition of subcutaneous daratumumab to induction, consolidation, and maintenance therapy improved progression-free survival.*

Triplet therapy with bortezomib, lenalidomide, and dexamethasone (VRd), followed by autologous stem-cell transplant (ASCT) and lenalidomide maintenance is a standard of care for transplant-eligible myeloma patients. Investigators now report a multicenter, phase 3 trial comparing VRd to VRd plus the anti-CD38 antibody daratumumab (D-VRd) administered subcutaneously (1800 mg) with induction (4 cycles), post-ASCT consolidation (2 cycles), and lenalidomide maintenance therapy until disease progression.

A total of 709 transplant-eligible patients aged 18–70 years were randomized. At a median follow-up of 48 months, the primary endpoint — progression-free survival (PFS) — was significantly better in the D-VRd group (hazard ratio for disease progression or death, 0.42). Estimated PFS rates were 84% in the D-VRd group versus 68% in the VRd group. Two key secondary endpoints — complete response or better and minimal residual disease (MRD)–negative status — also favored D-VRd. Data on overall survival were immature.

The most common grade 3 or 4 adverse events in the D-VRd and VRd groups included neutropenia (62% and 51%, respectively) and thrombocytopenia (29% and 17%). Serious adverse events occurred in 57% of the D-VRd group and 49% of the VRd group, and adverse events leading to treatment discontinuation occurred in 9% and 21%, respectively.

The addition of the anti-CD38 monoclonal antibody daratumumab to VRd induction, post-ASCT consolidation, and maintenance lenalidomide significantly improved the complete response rate, the achievement of negative MRD status, and PFS. Longer follow-up is needed to assess any improvement in overall survival.

## Belantamab Mafodotin, Bortezomib, and Dexamethasone for Multiple Myeloma[74]

*Belantamab mafodotin had single-agent activity in patients with relapsed or refractory multiple myeloma, a finding that supports further evaluation of the agent in combination with standard-of-care therapies.*

In this phase 3, open-label, randomized trial, researchers evaluated belantamab mafodotin, bortezomib, and dexamethasone (BVd), as compared with daratumumab, bortezomib, and dexamethasone (DVd), in patients who had progression of multiple myeloma after at least one line of therapy. The primary end point was progression-free survival. Key secondary end points were overall survival, response duration, and minimal residual disease (MRD)–negative status.

Belantamab mafodotin is a humanized IgG1κ monoclonal antibody against the B-cell maturation antigen (BCMA) conjugated with a cytotoxic agent, maleimidocaproyl monomethyl auristatin F. The antibody-drug conjugate binds to BCMA on myeloma cell surfaces causing cell cycle arrest and inducing antibody-dependent cellular cytotoxicity.

In total, 494 patients were randomly assigned to receive BVd (243 patients) or DVd (251 patients). At a median follow-up of 28.2 months (range, 0.1 to 40.0), median progression-free survival was 36.6 months in the BVd group and 13.4 months in the DVd group ($p<0.001$). Overall survival at 18 months was 84% in the BVd group and 73% in the DVd group. An analysis of the restricted mean response duration favored BVd over DVd ($p<0.001$). A complete response plus MRD-negative status occurred in 25% of the patients in the BVd group and 10% of those in the DVd group. Grade 3 or higher adverse events occurred in 95% of the patients in the BVd group and 78% of those in the DVd group. Ocular events were more common in the BVd group than in the DVd group (79% vs. 29%); such events were managed with dose modifications, and events of worsening visual acuity mostly resolved.

As compared with DVd therapy, BVd therapy conferred a significant benefit with respect to progression-free survival among patients who had relapsed or refractory multiple myeloma after at least one line of therapy. Most patients had grade 3 or higher adverse events.

This interim analysis of the trial showed significantly better progression-free survival and a greater depth of response with the use of belantamab mafodotin combined with bortezomib and dexamethasone (BVd) than with daratumamab plus the same backbone regimen (DVd). Median progression-free survival was 36.6 months with BVd and 13.4 months with DVd (p<0.001). A trend toward a benefit with respect to overall survival was observed in the BVd group, but longer follow-up is required to determine significance. More grade 3 or higher adverse events were observed in the BVd group; however, the overall safety profile was as expected for the individual agents in the combination.

- **Belantamab Mafodotin, Pomalidomide, and Dexamethasone in Multiple Myeloma[114]**

*Progression-free survival among lenalidomide-exposed patients with relapsed or refractory myeloma was improved with BPd compared to PVd.*

Triplet or quadruplet therapies incorporating proteasome inhibitors, immunomodulators, and anti-CD38 antibodies have led to prolonged survival among patients with newly diagnosed multiple myeloma; however, most patients have a relapse. Frontline lenalidomide therapy has increased the number of patients with lenalidomide-refractory disease at the time of the first relapse.

In this phase 3, randomized, open-label trial, investigators evaluated belantamab mafodotin, pomalidomide, and dexamethasone (BPd), as compared with pomalidomide, bortezomib, and dexamethasone (PVd), in lenalidomide-exposed patients who had relapsed or refractory myeloma after at least one line of therapy. The primary end point was progression-free survival. Disease response and safety were also assessed.

A total of 302 patients underwent randomization; 155 were assigned to the BPd group, and 147 to the PVd group. At a median follow-up of 21.8 months (range, <0.1

to 39.2), the 12-month estimated progression-free survival with BPd was 71% compared with 51% with PVd ($p<0.001$). Grade 3 or higher adverse events occurred in 94% of the patients in the BPd group and 76% of those in the PVd group. Ocular events occurred in 89% of the patients who received BPd (grade 3 or 4 in 43%) and 30% of those who received PVd (grade 3 or 4 in 2%); ocular events in the BPd group were managed with belantamab mafodotin dose modification. Ocular events led to treatment discontinuation in 9% of the patients in the BPd group but in no patients in the PVd group.

Among lenalidomide-exposed patients with relapsed or refractory myeloma, BPd conferred a significantly greater benefit than PVd with respect to progression-free survival, as well as deeper, more durable responses. Ocular events were common but were controllable by belantamab mafodotin dose modification.

- **Quadruplet Therapy with Isatuximab for Newly Diagnosed Multiple Myeloma[103]**

*Adding this anti-CD38 monoclonal antibody to bortezomib, lenalidomide, and dexamethasone improved outcomes in patients ineligible for transplantation.*

Combining bortezomib, lenalidomide, and dexamethasone (VRd) is a well-established frontline therapy for treating multiple myeloma. Investigators now report long-term follow-up of a phase 3, multicenter trial that randomized 446 transplant-ineligible patients with multiple myeloma to VRd plus isatuximab (isa-VRd) or VRd alone.

Patients (age range 18–80) had previously untreated disease and were ineligible for transplantation due to age over 65 or significant comorbidities. Four 6-week induction cycles in each study arm were followed by continuous 4-week maintenance cycles of isa-Rd or Rd. For 25 patients receiving Rd whose disease progressed, crossover to isa-Rd was permitted. The median follow-up was 59.7 months.

The 60-month progression-free survival was significantly greater with isa-VRd than VRd alone (63.2% vs. 45.2%; hazard ratio, 0.60). Achievement of complete remission was significantly greater with isa-VRd than VRd-only (75% vs. 61%); this was also true for minimal residual disease (MRD)–negative status (58% vs. 44%, respectively).

## CHAPTER 25. POLYCYTHEMIA VERA

- **Reducing Therapeutic Phlebotomy in Polycythemia Vera[51]**

*A hepcidin mimetic, rusfertide, was effective in maintaining hematocrit <45% with minimal or no phlebotomies.*

Treatment for polycythemia vera is based on phlebotomy and induction of iron deficiency to maintain a hematocrit <45% and aspirin to reduce risk for thromboembolic events; many patients are also given cytoreductive hydroxyurea, JAK2 inhibitors, or interferon alfa. In a phase 2 trial, investigators tested the efficacy and safety of rusfertide, a peptide mimetic of endogenous hepcidin that induces functional iron deficiency and decreases erythropoiesis.

In part 1 of the study, 70 patients with phlebotomy-dependent disease received a 28-week dose-finding course of weekly subcutaneous rusfertide administered at 10 to 120 mg, dosed to maintain a hematocrit <45%. During part 2 of the study, 59 patients were randomized to a 12-week double-blind course of continued rusfertide or placebo. In the ongoing part 3, all patients are receiving rusfertide up to year 3. Patients could continue prior cytoreductive treatment during the study.

The mean baseline phlebotomy rate was 8.7 per year, which decreased to 0.6 per year during part 1 of the study. In part 2, an ongoing response (the primary endpoint) occurred in 60% of patients randomized to rusfertide versus 17% randomized to placebo (P=0.002). Serum ferritin levels increased while patients were on rusfertide. Patient-reported symptoms improved with rusfertide treatment; 10 grade 3 adverse events occurred, and 4 patients discontinued treatment.

Rusfertide represents a novel approach to maintaining a hematocrit <45% without periodic phlebotomy and shows promising early benefit for systemic symptoms. Adverse events did not increase in patients who continued cytoreductive therapy.

# CHAPTER 26. MYELODYSPLASIA

- **Reducing Red Blood Cell Transfusions in Lower-Risk Myelodysplastic Syndromes[108]**

*First-line treatment with luspatercept, compared with erythropoietin alfa, significantly improved anemia and reduced the need for RBC transfusions in adults with very-low, low, and intermediate-risk MDS. Luspatercept is a recombinant fusion protein that binds TGF-β superfamily ligands, inhibits aberrant signaling, and enhances erythroid maturation and differentiation.*

Investigators reported the final analysis of a multinational, open-label, phase 3 trial (COMMANDS) comparing luspatercept to erythropoietin alfa in transfusion-dependent patients with very low, low, or intermediate risk MDS (as defined by the Revised International Prognostic Scoring System). Patients who had not received prior erythropoiesis-stimulating agents (ESA) were randomized to subcutaneous luspatercept (1 mg/kg titrated up to 1.75 mg/kg, once every 3 weeks) or subcutaneous erythropoietin alfa (450 IU/kg titrated up to 1050 IU/kg once per week) for at least 24 weeks.

With a median follow-up of 17 months, the primary endpoint - independence from RBC transfusion for 12 or more weeks plus a mean hemoglobin increase of at least 1.5 g/dL within the first 24 weeks - was achieved by 110/182 (60%) of the luspatercept group versus 63/181 (35%) of the erythropoietin alfa group ($p<0.0001$). Higher luspatercept responses were observed in patients with SF3B1 mutations, positive ring sideroblast MDS subtype, lower baseline transfusion requirements (<4 units per 8 weeks), and serum erythropoietin levels <200 U/L. Fatigue, dyspnea, and thromboembolic events were more frequent with luspatercept; 13% of luspatercept recipients discontinued therapy due to treatment-related adverse events, versus 9% with erythropoietin alfa. Rates of progression to high-risk MDS or acute myeloid leukemia were low and did not differ between study arms.

# CHAPTER 27. OTHER DEVELOPMENTS IN CANCER MEDICINE

- **Ponsegromab for the Treatment of Cancer Cachexia[78]**

*In patients with cancer cachexia and elevated growth differentiation factor (GDF)-15 serum levels, the inhibition of GDF-15 with the monoclonal antibody ponsegromab resulted in increased weight gain and overall activity level and reduced cachexia symptoms.*

The investigators performed a phase 2, randomized, double-blind, 12-week trial in patients with cancer cachexia and an elevated serum GDF-15 level (≥1500 pg per milliliter) in a 1:1:1:1 ratio to receive ponsegromab at a dose of 100 mg, 200 mg, or 400 mg or to receive placebo, administered subcutaneously every 4 weeks for three doses.

The inhibition of GDF-15 with ponsegromab resulted in increased weight gain at each dose level of ponsegromab and increased appetite, increased overall activity level and reduced cachexia symptoms in the group receiving the 400 mg dose of ponsegromab compared to placebo. These findings confirmed that GDF-15 is a driver of cachexia in malignant disease.

- **Axatilimab in Recurrent or Refractory Chronic Graft-versus-Host Disease[82]**

*Targeting CSF1R-dependent monocytes and macrophages with axatilimab resulted in a high incidence of response among patients with recurrent or refractory chronic graft-versus-host disease after allogeneic hematopoietic stem cell transplantation*

In a phase 2, multinational, randomized study, the investigators evaluated axatilimab, a colony-stimulating factor 1 receptor (CSF-1R) blocking monoclonal antibody, at three different doses in patients with recurrent or refractory chronic GVHD:

1. 0.3 mg per kilogram of body weight every 2 weeks
2. 1 mg per kilogram every 2 weeks
3. 3 mg per kilogram every 4 weeks.

An overall response was observed in 74% of the patients in the 0.3-mg dose group, 67% of the patients in the 1-mg dose group, and 50% of the patients in the 3-mg dose group.

- **T-Cell Lymphoma Following CAR T-Cell Therapy[100,101,102]**

*Occurrence of this second malignancy is rare after CAR T cell therapy, but awareness of it is essential for patients and the oncology care team. Fully understanding the molecular mechanisms of such an event is also vital. Cellular immunotherapy with chimeric antigen receptor (CAR) T-cell products can provide durable responses in relapsed and refractory B-cell malignancies, but rare cases of T-cell malignancy among patients treated with CAR T have been identified. Reports of secondary T-cell malignancies in CAR-T–treated patients led to a "black-box warning" from the U.S. Food and Drug Administration for commercial CAR-T products. Approximately 20 to 25 T-cell lymphoma cases have been reported in more than 34,000 CAR-T therapy recipients.*

To assess the risk of second primary malignancies in recipients of CAR-T therapy, investigators conducted a single-institution retrospective analysis. Since 2016 the study cohort consisted of 724 patients who underwent 791 therapeutic CAR-T infusions. A single case of a T-cell lymphoma positive for Epstein-Barr virus was identified in a 59-year-old woman previously treated with CAR T-cell therapy (axicabtagene ciloleucel) for relapsed diffuse large B-cell lymphoma. Detailed molecular analysis showed that the two lymphomas were distinct, although a pre-existing T-cell clonal population was found in blood samples obtained prior to CAR T administration. The T-cell lymphoma was not derived from the CAR T-cell population itself; additionally, CAR T retroviral vector integration was not identified in the T-cell lymphoma.

In a separate case report, a patient with myeloma treated with ciltacabtagene autoleucel (age 71) was later diagnosed with indolent T-cell lymphoma. Lentiviral insertion in tumor DNA was found in addition to other potentially transforming mutations.

Active reporting of these cases will be essential to understanding the true incidence and associated risk factors. Detailed molecular analysis of mechanisms, as in these two studies, will be highly informative.

- **Distal DVTs Are High Risk in Patients with Cancer[40]**

*Distal and proximal deep venous thrombosis were associated with similar outcomes in patients with cancer.*

Patients without cancer who develop distal deep venous thrombosis (DVT) of the leg (i.e., calf DVT) have lower risk for developing recurrent venous thromboembolism (VTE) than do patients with proximal DVT; whether the same is true for patients with cancer is unclear. Researchers used a 10-year international cohort of 110,000 patients with new DVTs to compare outcomes among patients with active cancer who developed distal DVT, patients with cancer who developed proximal DVT, and patients *without* cancer who developed distal DVT. Nearly all patients in each group received anticoagulation for at least 3 months, and outcomes were assessed at 3 and 12 months.

In patients with active cancer, three adverse outcomes — all-cause mortality, VTE recurrence, and major bleeding — were not significantly different in patients with distal DVT and in those with proximal DVT. However, patients *without* cancer who had distal DVT had adverse outcomes significantly less commonly than did patients with cancer who had distal DVT.

This study demonstrates that distal DVT in patients with cancer is associated with worse outcomes than in patients without cancer. The other key finding — similar incidences of adverse outcomes following distal DVT and proximal DVT in patients with cancer — suggests that distal DVT should not be considered a less serious complication in this patient population.

- **A Next-Generation Version of the Multitarget Stool DNA Test (Cologuard)[45]**

*The new test appears to have similar sensitivity and higher specificity than its predecessor.*

Performance of the new version was examined in 20,000 people who were undergoing screening colonoscopy.

In 2014 a multitarget stool DNA test (Cologuard) was approved in the U.S.A. for colorectal cancer screening, based on a study that established the test's sensitivity and specificit. Now, industry-sponsored researchers present results of a study of a next generation stool DNA test, which contains more-recently identified markers of colorectal neoplasia plus a test for fecal hemoglobin.

About 20,000 asymptomatic adults (mean age, 63) had stool specimens analyzed by the next-generation test and by a commercial fecal immunochemical (FIT) test for comparison; all participants then underwent colonoscopy. Colonoscopy identified colorectal cancer in 98 people and advanced precancerous lesions (but not cancer) in 2,144 people. Findings for the next-generation test were as follows:

- Sensitivity was 94% for colorectal cancer and 43% for advanced precancerous lesions.
- Specificity (the proportion of people *without* cancer or advanced precancerous lesions whose test was negative) was 91%.
- Positive predictive value (the proportion of positive tests that were true positives for cancer or advanced neoplasia) was 38%.
- Negative predictive value (the proportion of negative tests that were true negatives for cancer or advanced neoplasia) was 93%.
- The stool DNA test was substantially more sensitive than FIT (94% vs. 67% for cancer; 43% vs. 23% for advanced precancerous lesions), but slightly less specific.

The new test appears to have similar sensitivity and higher specificity than its predecessor - which means fewer false positives.

- **Radiation Therapy for Asymptomatic Bone Metastases**[52]

  *Prophylactic radiation to asymptomatic, high-risk bone metastases reduced skeletal-related events and hospitalizations.*

Skeletal-related events (SREs) in patients with cancer metastases to bone can be reduced by 10% to 20% with bone-modifying agents such as bisphosphonates. Although radiation therapy is used to palliate painful bone metastases, data regarding its use in the asymptomatic setting are limited.

In this multicenter, phase 2 clinical trial, investigators compared prophylactic radiation therapy against standard of care for high-risk, asymptomatic bone metastases. Seventy-eight adults with widely metastatic solid tumor malignancies and 122 bone metastases were randomized to receive radiation therapy or standard of care (systemic therapy or observation). The most common primary cancers were lung (27%), breast (24%), and prostate (22%). The trial's primary outcome was SREs, defined as pathologic fracture, spinal cord compression, orthopedic surgery, or palliative radiation therapy for pain.

The radiation therapy arm had a significant reduction in SREs compared with the standard care arm (1.6% vs. 28.6%; $p<.001$). Additionally, significantly fewer patients in the radiation arm were hospitalized for SREs (0 vs. 11%, respectively; $p=.045$). Overall survival was longer in the radiation arm than the standard care arm (median, 1.7 vs. 1.0 years; hazard ratio, 0.49; $p=0.18$), but the study was not powered for this outcome. Among patients who were not on an opioid at study entry, opioid-free probability did not differ between arms (HR, 0.57; $P=0.5$). Treatment-related complications were uncommon, and no grade 3 or higher radiation-related adverse events were reported.

Prophylactic radiation therapy should be considered for asymptomatic, high-risk bone metastases in patients with widely metastatic solid tumor malignancies to help reduce SREs and hospitalization.

- **Risk Factors for Death After Neurologic Immune-Related Adverse Events**[57]

*In patients taking immune checkpoint inhibitors, noninflammatory encephalopathy and a myocarditis/myasthenia/myositis overlap syndrome were associated with highest mortality risk.*

Recent cohort studies have demonstrated that neurologic immune-related adverse events (nirAEs) following immune checkpoint inhibitor (ICI) therapy for cancer are frequent, varied, and associated with higher overall survival. Researchers conducted a retrospective cohort study of consecutive patients referred to a tertiary center during a 5-year period to characterize the clinical features of nirAEs and identify predictors of ICI response and survival.

The researchers identified 64 patients with confirmed nirAEs, 81% involving the central nervous system (CNS). The vast majority of CNS nirAE patients had encephalopathy, of which 73% were neither seropositive for well-characterized neural autoantibodies, nor had a distinctive encephalitis syndrome, nor had evidence of CNS inflammatory changes. The most common peripheral nervous system (PNS) syndrome was myasthenia and myositis (with or without myocarditis) overlap syndrome. Steroids were given to 91% of nirAE patients after a median of 90 days of symptoms, and 48% received additional immunotherapy. At 1-month follow-up, 72% of nirAE patients showed improvement, 9% had worsened, and 17% had died. Among the 53 patients who survived the first month, median follow-up was 6 months; during follow-up, 30% died, most commonly of cancer progression or cancer-related complications. Death was associated with lung cancer (hazard ratio, 2.5), encephalopathy without CNS inflammatory changes (HR, 5.0), and myasthenia/myositis/myocarditis overlap syndrome (HR, 6.6).

In this series of patients with nirAEs, a higher risk for death was seen in patients with encephalopathy without CNS inflammatory changes and in those with myasthenia/ myositis/myocarditis overlap syndrome. Most patient deaths occurred during the first month following symptom onset, suggesting the importance of early immunotherapy for nirAEs.

- **Primary VTE Prevention for Patients with Cancer**[70,71]

*In a randomized trial, primary prophylaxis in high-risk patients with lung or gastrointestinal cancers lowered incidence of thromboembolism.*

Based on results from randomized trials, current guidelines recommend primary prophylaxis against venous thromboembolism (VTE) for high-risk outpatients with cancer. However, few ambulatory patients with cancer receive VTE prophylaxis. Australian investigators identified 200 high-risk outpatients - defined as those with either elevated fibrinogen or D-dimer levels - who were being treated for gastrointestinal (GI) or lung cancer and randomized them to receive either low-molecular-weight heparin (LMWH) VTE prophylaxis or no prophylaxis. In addition, 128 low-risk patients (without elevation of fibrinogen or D-dimer) were followed in a low-risk observational arm.

In the randomized comparison between LMWH and no LMWH among high-risk patients, the LMWH group had significantly fewer thromboembolic events (8% vs. 23%) and significantly lower 6-month mortality (13% vs. 26%). In the low-risk observational cohort, thromboembolism occurred in 8% of patients, and 6-month mortality was 7%. Bleeding was uncommon (<2%) and not different among groups.

This study adds to the evidence showing that high-risk outpatients with lung or GI cancer — when appropriately risk stratified — can benefit substantially from pharmacologic VTE prophylaxis. Risk stratification in this trial was done with D-dimer and fibrinogen levels, but other validated tools also are available (e.g., the Khorana Risk Score). Despite lack of blinding, this study should persuade physicians to provide VTE prophylaxis to high-risk outpatients with cancer. Direct-acting oral anticoagulants are an acceptable alternative to LMWH.

## CONCLUSIONS

Predictably, most new treatment approaches described in the peer-reviewed medical literature during the period January 2024 to October 2024 involved the four commonest cancers – carcinoma of the lung, carcinoma of the breast, colo-rectal carcinoma and carcinoma of the prostate. There were also many innovative advances in non-Hodgkin lymphoma and myeloma.

Happily, there were also treatments described for diseases which have not had active treatments available up until now (other than surgery in selected patients). Examples include pancreatic carcinoma, hepatocellular carcinoma, biliary tract neoplasms and neuroendocrine tumors. On the other hand, some diseases were notable for their absence from this book – for example, brain tumors, mesothelioma and sarcomas.

Many of the new treatments involved the application of immune checkpoint inhibitors and tyrosine kinase inhibitors. The status of medical oncology is almost unrecognizable from its nascent development in the 1960s and 1970s. It is developing very rapidly now and likely will continue to do so in the coming years.

## REFERENCES

1. Zhou C, Tang KJ, Cho BC, Liu B, Paz-Ares L, Cheng S, Kitazono S, Thiagarajan M, Goldman JW, Sabari JK, Sanborn RE, Mansfield AS, Hung JY, Boyer M, Popat S, Mourão Dias J, Felip E, Majem M, Gumus M, Kim SW, Ono A, Xie J, Bhattacharya A, Agrawal T, Shreeve SM, Knoblauch RE, Park K, Girard N; PAPILLON Investigators. Amivantamab plus Chemotherapy in NSCLC with EGFR Exon 20 Insertions. N Engl J Med. 2023 Nov 30;389(22):2039-2051. doi: 10.1056/NEJMoa2306441. Epub 2023 Oct 21. PMID: 37870976.

2. Lu S, Kato T, Dong X, Ahn MJ, Quang LV, Soparattanapaisarn N, Inoue T, Wang CL, Huang M, Yang JC, Cobo M, Özgüroğlu M, Casarini I, Khiem DV, Sriuranpong V, Cronemberger E, Takahashi T, Runglodvatana Y, Chen M, Huang X, Grainger E, Ghiorghiu D, van der Gronde T, Ramalingam SS; LAURA Trial Investigators. Osimertinib after Chemoradiotherapy in Stage III EGFR-Mutated NSCLC. N Engl J Med. 2024 Jun 2. doi: 10.1056/NEJMoa2402614. Epub ahead of print. PMID: 38828946.

3. Hochhaus A, Wang J, Kim DW, Kim DDH, Mayer J, Goh YT, le Coutre P, Takahashi N, Kim I, Etienne G, Andorsky D, Issa GC, Larson RA, Bombaci F, Kapoor S, McCulloch T, Malek K, Yau L, Ifrah S, Hoch M, Cortes JE, Hughes TP; ASC4FIRST Investigators. Asciminib in Newly Diagnosed Chronic Myeloid Leukemia. N Engl J Med. 2024 May 31. doi: 10.1056/NEJMoa2400858. Epub ahead of print. PMID: 38820078.

4. Litzow MR et al. Blinatumomab for MRD-negative acute lymphoblastic leukemia in adults. N Engl J Med 2024 Jul 25; 391:320. (https://doi.org/10.1056/NEJMoa2312948)

5. Liu X, Zhang Y, Yang KY, Zhang N, Jin F, Zou GR, Zhu XD, Xie FY, Liang XY, Li WF, He ZY, Chen NY, Hu WH, Wu HJ, Shi M, Zhou GQ, Mao YP, Guo R, Sun R, Huang J, Liang SQ, Wu WL, Su Z, Li L, Ai P, He YX, Zang J, Chen L, Lin L, Huang SH, Xu C, Lv JW, Li YQ, Hong SB, Jie YS, Li H, Huang SW, Liang YL, Wang YQ, Peng YL, Zhu JH, Zang SB, Liu SR, Lin QG, Li HJ, Tian L, Liu LZ, Zhao HY, Lin AH, Li JB, Liu N, Tang LL, Chen YP, Sun Y, Ma J. Induction-concurrent chemoradiotherapy with or without sintilimab in patients with locoregionally advanced nasopharyngeal carcinoma in China (CONTINUUM): a multicentre, open-label, parallel-group, randomised, controlled, phase 3 trial. Lancet. 2024 Jun 22;403(10445):2720-2731. doi: 10.1016/S0140-6736(24)00594-4. Epub 2024 May 30. PMID: 38824941.

6. Singh S et al. [$^{177}$Lu]Lu-DOTA-TATE plus long-acting octreotide versus high–dose long-acting octreotide for the treatment of newly diagnosed, advanced grade 2–3, well-differentiated, gastroenteropancreatic neuroendocrine tumours (NETTER-2): An open-label, randomised, phase 3 study. Lancet 2024 Jun 29; 403:2807. (https://doi.org/10.1016/S0140-6736(24)00701-3)

7. Melani C et al. Combination targeted therapy in relapsed diffuse large B-cell lymphoma. N Engl J Med 2024 Jun 20; 390:2143. (https://doi.org/10.1056/NEJMoa2401532)

8. Qiu M-Z et al. Tislelizumab plus chemotherapy versus placebo plus chemotherapy as first line treatment for advanced gastric or gastro-oesophageal junction adenocarcinoma: RATIONALE-305 randomised, double blind, phase 3 trial. BMJ 2024 May 28; 385:e078876. (https://doi.org/10.1136/bmj-2023-078876)

9. Long GV et al. Final results for adjuvant dabrafenib plus trametinib in stage III melanoma. N Engl J Med 2024 Jun 19; [e-pub]. (https://doi.org/10.1056/NEJMoa2404139)

10. Chalabi M et al. Neoadjuvant immunotherapy in locally advanced mismatch repair–deficient colon cancer. N Engl J Med 2024 Jun 6; 390:1949. (https://doi.org/10.1056/NEJMoa2400634)

11. Blank CU et al. Neoadjuvant nivolumab and ipilimumab in resectable stage III melanoma. N Engl J Med 2024 Jun 2; [e-pub]. (https://doi.org/10.1056/NEJMoa2402604).

12. Pérez-García JM et al. 3-year invasive disease-free survival with chemotherapy de-escalation using an 18F-FDG-PET-based, pathological complete response-adapted strategy in HER2-positive early breast cancer (PHERGain): A randomised, open-label, phase 2 trial. Lancet 2024 Apr 27; 403:1649. (https://doi.org/10.1016/S0140-6736(24)00054-0)

13. Vauthey JN et al. Chemotherapy regimen predicts steatohepatitis and an increase in 90-day mortality after surgery for hepatic colorectal metastases. J Clin Oncol 2006 May 1; 24:2065-72.

14. Pinto C et al. Fluorouracil, leucovorin, and irinotecan plus cetuximab versus cetuximab as maintenance therapy in first-line therapy for RAS and BRAF wild-type metastatic colorectal cancer: Phase III ERMES study. J Clin Oncol 2024 Apr 10; 42:1278. (https://doi.org/10.1200/JCO.23.01021)

15. Newcomb LF et al. Long-term outcomes in patients using protocol-directed active surveillance for prostate cancer. JAMA 2024 May 30; [e-pub]. (https://doi.org/10.1001/jama.2024.6695)

16. Parker CC et al. Adding 6 months of androgen deprivation therapy to postoperative radiotherapy for prostate cancer: A comparison of short-course versus no androgen deprivation therapy in the RADICALS-HD randomised controlled trial. Lancet 2024 Jun 1; 403:2405. (https://doi.org/10.1016/S0140-6736(24)00548-8)

17. Dreyling M et al. Ibrutinib combined with immunochemotherapy with or without autologous stem-cell transplantation versus immunochemotherapy and autologous stem-cell transplantation in previously untreated patients with mantle cell lymphoma (TRIANGLE): A three-arm, randomised, open-label, phase 3 superiority trial of the European Mantle Cell Lymphoma Network. Lancet 2024 May 25; 403:2293. (https://doi.org/10.1016/S0140-6736(24)00184-3)

18. Martin P and Maddocks K. Does TRIANGLE take down transplantation in mantle cell lymphoma? Lancet 2024 May 25; 403:2264. (https://doi.org/10.1016/S0140-6736(24)00301-5)

19. Cascone T et al. Perioperative nivolumab in resectable lung cancer. N Engl J Med 2024 May 16; 390:1756. (https://doi.org/10.1056/NEJMoa2311926)

20. Hu Y et al. Sequential CD7 CAR T-cell therapy and allogeneic HSCT without GVHD prophylaxis. N Engl J Med 2024 Apr 25; 390:1467. (https://doi.org/10.1056/NEJMoa2313812)

21. Blaise D. CAR as booster to launch allogeneic transplantation in refractory leukemia. N Engl J Med 2024 Apr 25; 390:1526. (https://doi.org/10.1056/NEJMe2403003)

22. Wang M et al. Lisocabtagene maraleucel in relapsed/refractory mantle cell lymphoma: Primary analysis of the mantle cell lymphoma cohort from TRANSCEND NHL 001, a phase I multicenter seamless design study. J Clin Oncol 2024 Apr 1; 42:1146. (https://doi.org/10.1200/JCO.23.02214)

23. Kim S et al. Atezolizumab plus modified docetaxel, cisplatin, and fluorouracil as first-line treatment for advanced anal cancer (SCARCE C17-02 PRODIGE 60): A randomised, non-comparative, phase 2 study. Lancet Oncol 2024 Apr; 25:518. (https://doi.org/10.1016/S1470-2045(24)00081-0)

24. Hu H et al. Neoadjuvant chemotherapy with oxaliplatin and fluoropyrimidine versus upfront surgery for locally advanced colon cancer: The randomized, phase III OPTICAL trial. *J Clin Oncol* 2021 Apr 2; [e-pub]. (https://doi.org/10.1200/JCO.23.01889)

25. Garraway IP et al. Prostate Cancer Foundation screening guidelines for Black men in the United States. NEJM Evid 2024 May; 3:EVIDoa2300289. (https://doi.org/10.1056/EVIDoa2300289)

26. Budde LE et al. Durable responses with mosunetuzumab in relapsed/refractory indolent and aggressive B-cell non-Hodgkin lymphomas: Extended follow-up of a phase I/II study. J Clin Oncol 2024 Mar 28; [e-pub]. (https://doi.org/10.1200/JCO.23.02329)

27. US Preventive Services Task Force. Screening for breast cancer: US Preventive Services Task Force recommendation statement. JAMA 2024 Apr 30; [e-pub]. (https://doi.org/10.1001/jama.2024.5534)

28. Henderson JT et al. Screening for breast cancer: Evidence report and systematic review for the US Preventive Services Task Force. JAMA 2024 Apr 30; [e-pub]. (https://doi.org/10.1001/jama.2023.25844)

29. Trentham-Dietz A et al. Collaborative modeling to compare different breast cancer screening strategies: A decision analysis for the US Preventive Services Task Force. JAMA 2024 Apr 30; [e-pub]. (https://doi.org/10.1001/jama.2023.24766)

30. Wu Y-L et al. Alectinib in resected ALK-positive non–small-cell lung cancer. N Engl J Med 2024 Apr 11; 390:1265. (https://doi.org/10.1056/NEJMoa2310532)

31. Leon-Ferre RA et al. Tumor-infiltrating lymphocytes in triple-negative breast cancer. JAMA 2024 Apr 2; 331:1135. (https://doi.org/10.1001/jama.2024.3056)

32. de Boniface J et al. Omitting axillary dissection in breast cancer with sentinel-node metastases. N Engl J Med 2024 Apr 4; 390:1163. (https://doi.org/10.1056/NEJMoa2313487)

33. Rahbari NN et al. Primary tumor resection before systemic therapy in patients with colon cancer and unresectable metastases: Combined results of the SYNCHRONOUS and CCRe-IV trials. J Clin Oncol 2024 Feb 27; [e-pub]. (https://doi.org/10.1200/JCO.23.01540)

34. Lorusso D et al. Pembrolizumab or placebo with chemoradiotherapy followed by pembrolizumab or placebo for newly diagnosed, high-risk, locally advanced cervical cancer (ENGOT-cx11/GOG-3047/KEYNOTE-A18): A randomised, double-blind, phase 3 clinical trial. Lancet 2024 Apr 6; 403:1341. (https://doi.org/10.1016/S0140-6736(24)00317-9)

35. Hamidi S et al. Checkpoint inhibition in addition to dabrafenib/trametinib for BRAFV600E-mutated anaplastic thyroid carcinoma. Thyroid 2024 Mar; 34:336; [e-pub]. (https://doi.org/10.1089/thy.2023.0573)

36. Slamon D et al. Ribociclib plus endocrine therapy in early breast cancer. N Engl J Med 2024 Mar 21; 390:1080. (https://doi.org/10.1056/NEJMoa2305488)

37. Eythorsson E et al. Development of a multivariable model to predict the need for bone marrow sampling in persons with monoclonal gammopathy of undetermined significance: A cohort study nested in a clinical trial. *Ann Intern Med* 2024 Apr; 177:449. (https://doi.org/10.7326/M23-2540)

38. Schorb E et al. High-dose chemotherapy and autologous haematopoietic stem-cell transplantation in older, fit patients with primary diffuse large B-cell CNS lymphoma (MARTA): A single-arm, phase 2 trial. Lancet Haematol 2024 Mar; 11:e196. (https://doi.org/10.1016/S2352-3026(23)00371-X)

39. Mahadeo KM et al. Tabelecleucel for allogeneic haematopoietic stem-cell or solid organ transplant recipients with Epstein–Barr virus-positive post-transplant lymphoproliferative disease after failure of rituximab or rituximab and chemotherapy (ALLELE): A phase 3, multicentre, open-label trial. Lancet Oncol 2024 Mar; 25:376. (https://doi.org/10.1016/S1470-2045(23)00649-6)

40. Galanaud J-P et al. Clinical presentation and outcomes of patients with cancer-associated isolated distal deep vein thrombosis. J Clin Oncol 2024 Feb 10; 42:529. (https://doi.org/10.1200/JCO.23.00429)

41. Palmieri C et al. Activity and safety of enobosarm, a novel, oral, selective androgen receptor modulator, in androgen receptor-positive, oestrogen receptor-positive, and HER2-negative advanced breast cancer (Study G200802): A

randomised, open-label, multicentre, multinational, parallel design, phase 2 trial. Lancet Oncol 2024 Mar; 25:317. (https://doi.org/10.1016/S1470-2045(24)00004-4)

42. Qin S et al. Nimotuzumab plus gemcitabine for K-Ras wild-type locally advanced or metastatic pancreatic cancer. J Clin Oncol 2023 Nov 20; 41:5163. (https://doi.org/10.1200/JCO.22.02630)

43. Chung DC et al. A cell-free DNA blood-based test for colorectal cancer screening. N Engl J Med 2024 Mar 14; 390:973. (https://doi.org/10.1056/NEJMoa2304714)

44. Carrato A et al. Nab-Paclitaxel plus Gemcitabine and FOLFOX in Metastatic Pancreatic Cancer. NEJM Evid 2024 Feb; 3:EVIDoa2300144. (https://doi.org/10.1056/EVIDoa2300144)

45. Imperiale TF et al. Next-generation multitarget stool DNA test for colorectal cancer screening. N Engl J Med 2024 Mar 14; 390:984. (https://doi.org/10.1056/NEJMoa2310336)

46. Pott C et al. Minimal residual disease status predicts outcome in patients with previously untreated follicular lymphoma: A prospective analysis of the phase III GALLIUM study. J Clin Oncol 2024 Feb 10; 42:550. (https://doi.org/10.1200/JCO.23.00838)

47. Powles T et al. Enfortumab vedotin and pembrolizumab in untreated advanced urothelial cancer. N Engl J Med 2024 Mar 7; 390:875. (https://doi.org/10.1056/NEJMoa2312117)

48. Niegisch G. Enfortumab vedotin and pembrolizumab — A new perspective on urothelial cancer. N Engl J Med 2024 Mar 7; 390:944. (https://doi.org/10.1056/NEJMe2400311)

49. Foà R et al. Long-term results of the dasatinib-blinatumomab protocol for adult Philadelphia-positive ALL. J Clin Oncol 2023 Dec 21; [e-pub]. (https://doi.org/10.1200/JCO.23.01075)

50. Plante M et al. Simple versus radical hysterectomy in women with low-risk cervical cancer. N Engl J Med 2024 Feb 29; 390:819. (https://doi.org/10.1056/NEJMoa2308900)

51. Kremyanskaya M et al. Rusfertide, a hepcidin mimetic, for control of erythrocytosis in polycythemia vera. N Engl J Med 2024 Feb 22; 390:723. (https://doi.org/10.1056/NEJMoa2308809)

52. Gillespie EF et al. Prophylactic radiation therapy versus standard of care for patients with high-risk asymptomatic bone metastases: A multicenter, randomized phase ii clinical trial. J Clin Oncol 2024 Jan 1; 42:38. (https://doi.org/10.1200/JCO.23.00753)

53. Ferrigno Guajardo AS et al. Taxanes for the treatment of breast cancer during pregnancy: An international cohort study. J Natl Cancer Inst 2024 Feb 8; 116:239. (https://doi.org/10.1093/jnci/djad219)

54. O'Sullivan CC and Ruddy KJ. Improving our treatment of breast cancer during pregnancy. J Natl Cancer Inst 2024 Feb 8; 116:183. (https://doi.org/10.1093/jnci/djad259)

55. Mannu GS et al. Invasive breast cancer and breast cancer death after non-screen detected ductal carcinoma in situ from 1990 to 2018 in England: Population based cohort study. BMJ 2024 Jan 24; 384:e075498. (https://doi.org/10.1136/bmj-2023-075498)

56. Narod SA et al. Breast cancer mortality after a diagnosis of ductal carcinoma in situ. JAMA Oncol 2015 Oct; 1:888. (https://doi.org/10.1001/jamaoncol.2015.2510)

57. Fonseca E et al. Neurological adverse events related to immune-checkpoint inhibitors in Spain: A retrospective cohort study. Lancet Neurol 2023 Dec; 22:1150. (https://doi.org/10.1016/S1474-4422(23)00335-6)

58. Lee NY et al. Hypoxia-directed treatment of human papillomavirus–related oropharyngeal carcinoma. J Clin Oncol 2024 Jan 19; [e-pub]. (https://doi.org/10.1200/JCO.23.01308)

59. Stelljes M et al. Inotuzumab ozogamicin as induction therapy for patients older than 55 years with Philadelphia chromosome–negative B-precursor ALL. J Clin Oncol 2024 Jan 20; 42:273. (https://doi.org/10.1200/JCO.23.00546)

60. Logan A. Innovating simpler and less toxic frontline management for adults with ALL. J Clin Oncol 2024 Jan 20; 42:250. (https://doi.org/10.1200/JCO.23.01726)

61. Al Hussein Al Awamlh B et al. Functional outcomes after localized prostate cancer treatment. JAMA 2024 Jan 23/30; 331:302. (https://doi.org/10.1001/jama.2023.26491)

62. Weber JS et al. Individualised neoantigen therapy mRNA-4157 (V940) plus pembrolizumab versus pembrolizumab monotherapy in resected melanoma (KEYNOTE-942): A randomised, phase 2b study. Lancet 2024 Jan 18; [e-pub]. (https://doi.org/10.1016/S0140-6736(23)02268-7)

63. Hoster E et al. Predictive value of minimal residual disease for efficacy of rituximab maintenance in mantle cell lymphoma: Results from the European Mantle Cell Lymphoma Elderly Trial. J Clin Oncol 2023 Nov 22; [e-pub]. (https://doi.org/10.1200/JCO.23.00899)

64. Rendle KA et al. Rates of downstream procedures and complications associated with lung cancer screening in routine clinical practice: A Retrospective Cohort Study. Ann Intern Med 2024 Jan; 177:18. (https://doi.org/10.7326/M23-0653)

65. Xu J et al. Sintilimab plus chemotherapy for unresectable gastric or gastroesophageal junction cancer: The ORIENT-16 randomized clinical trial. JAMA 2023 Dec 5; 330:2064. (https://doi.org/10.1001/jama.2023.19918)

66. Munir T et al. Chronic lymphocytic leukemia therapy guided by measurable residual disease. N Engl J Med 2023 Dec 10; [e-pub]. (https://doi.org/10.1056/NEJMoa2310063)

67. Drilon A et al. Repotrectinib in ROS1 fusion–positive non–small-cell lung cancer. N Engl J Med 2024 Jan 11; 390:118. (https://doi.org/10.1056/NEJMoa2302299)

68. Sonneveld P et al. Daratumumab, bortezomib, lenalidomide, and dexamethasone for multiple myeloma. N Engl J Med 2023 Dec 12; [e-pub]. (https://doi.org/10.1056/NEJMoa2312054)

69. Fizazi K et al. Targeted inhibition of CYP11A1 in castration-resistant prostate cancer NEJM Evid 2024 Jan; 3:EVIDoa2300171. (https://doi.org/10.1056/EVIDoa2300171)

70. Alexander M et al. Risk-directed ambulatory thromboprophylaxis in lung and gastrointestinal cancers: The TARGET-TP randomized clinical trial. JAMA Oncol 2023 Nov; 9:1536. (https://doi.org/10.1001/jamaoncol.2023.3634)

71. Khorana AA. Primary thromboprophylaxis in people with cancer — Where next? JAMA Oncol 2023 Nov; 9:1545. (https://doi.org/10.1001/jamaoncol.2023.3569)

72. Ryan CE et al. Germline CDH1 variants and lifetime cancer risk. JAMA 2024 Jun 14; [e-pub]. (https://doi.org/10.1001/jama.2024.10852)

73. Scherer LD et al. Mammography screening preferences among screening-eligible women in their 40s: A national U.S. survey. Ann Intern Med 2024 Jul 16; [e-pub]. (https://doi.org/10.7326/M23-3325)

74. Hungria, V et al. Belantamab Mafodotin, Bortezomib, and Dexamethasone for Multiple Myeloma. N Engl J Med 2024;391:461-462. DOI: 10.1056/NEJMe2406799

75. Vergote et al. Tisotumab Vedotin as Second- or Third-Line Therapy for Recurrent Cervical Cancer. N Engl J Med 2024; 391:44-55. DOI: 10.1056/NEJMoa2313811

76. Plotkin, SR et al. Brigatinib in NF2-Related Schwannomatosis with Progressive Tumors. N Engl J Med 2024;390:2284-2294. DOI: 10.1056/NEJMoa240098

77. Hugosson J, Godtman RA, Wallstrom J, Axcrona U, Bergh A, Egevad L, Geterud K, Khatami A, Socratous A, Spyratou V, Svensson L, Stranne J, Månsson M, Hellstrom M. Results after Four Years of Screening for Prostate Cancer with PSA and MRI. N Engl J Med. 2024 Sep 26;391(12):1083-1095. doi: 10.1056/NEJMoa2406050. PMID: 39321360.

78. Groarke JD, Crawford J, Collins SM, Lubaczewski S, Roeland EJ, Naito T, Hendifar AE, Fallon M, Takayama K, Asmis T, Dunne RF, Karahanoglu I, Northcott CA, Harrington MA, Rossulek M, Qiu R, Saxena AR. Ponsegromab for the Treatment of Cancer Cachexia. N Engl J Med. 2024 Sep 14. doi: 10.1056/NEJMoa2409515. Epub ahead of print. PMID: 39282907.

79. Chan JA, Geyer S, Zemla T, Knopp MV, Behr S, Pulsipher S, Ou FS, Dueck AC, Acoba J, Shergill A, Wolin EM, Halfdanarson TR, Konda B, Trikalinos NA, Tawfik B, Raj N, Shaheen S, Vijayvergia N, Dasari A, Strosberg JR, Kohn EC, Kulke MH, O'Reilly EM, Meyerhardt JA. Phase 3 Trial of Cabozantinib to Treat Advanced Neuroendocrine Tumors. N Engl J Med. 2024 Sep 16. doi: 10.1056/NEJMoa2403991. Epub ahead of print. PMID: 39282913.

80. Powles T, Catto JWF, Galsky MD, Al-Ahmadie H, Meeks JJ, Nishiyama H, Vu TQ, Antonuzzo L, Wiechno P, Atduev V, Kann AG, Kim TH, Suárez C, Chang CH, Roghmann F, Özgüroğlu M, Eigl BJ, Oliveira N, Buchler T, Gadot M, Zakharia Y, Armstrong J, Gupta A, Hois S, van der Heijden MS; NIAGARA Investigators. Perioperative Durvalumab with Neoadjuvant Chemotherapy in Operable Bladder Cancer. N Engl J Med. 2024 Sep 15. doi: 10.1056/NEJMoa2408154. Epub ahead of print. PMID: 39282910.

81. Cheng Y, Spigel DR, Cho BC, Laktionov KK, Fang J, Chen Y, Zenke Y, Lee KH, Wang Q, Navarro A, Bernabe R, Buchmeier EL, Chang JW, Shiraishi Y, Goksu SS, Badzio A, Shi A, Daniel DB, Hoa NTT, Zemanova M, Mann H, Gowda H, Jiang H, Senan S; ADRIATIC Investigators. Durvalumab after Chemoradiotherapy in Limited-Stage Small-Cell Lung

Cancer. N Engl J Med. 2024 Oct 10;391(14):1313-1327. doi: 10.1056/NEJMoa2404873. Epub 2024 Sep 13. PMID: 39268857.

82. Wolff D, Cutler C, Lee SJ, Pusic I, Bittencourt H, White J, Hamadani M, Arai S, Salhotra A, Perez-Simon JA, Alousi A, Choe H, Kwon M, Bermúdez A, Kim I, Socié G, Chhabra S, Radojcic V, O'Toole T, Tian C, Ordentlich P, DeFilipp Z, Kitko CL; AGAVE-201 Investigators. Axatilimab in Recurrent or Refractory Chronic Graft-versus-Host Disease. N Engl J Med. 2024 Sep 19;391(11):1002-1014. doi: 10.1056/NEJMoa2401537. PMID: 39292927.

83. Schmid P, Cortes J, Dent R, McArthur H, Pusztai L, Kümmel S, Denkert C, Park YH, Hui R, Harbeck N, Takahashi M, Im SA, Untch M, Fasching PA, Mouret-Reynier MA, Foukakis T, Ferreira M, Cardoso F, Zhou X, Karantza V, Tryfonidis K, Aktan G, O'Shaughnessy J; KEYNOTE-522 Investigators. Overall Survival with Pembrolizumab in Early-Stage Triple-Negative Breast Cancer. N Engl J Med. 2024 Sep 15. doi: 10.1056/NEJMoa2409932. Epub ahead of print. PMID: 39282906.

84. Bardia A, Hu X, Dent R, Yonemori K, Barrios CH, O'Shaughnessy JA, Wildiers H, Pierga JY, Zhang Q, Saura C, Biganzoli L, Sohn J, Im SA, Lévy C, Jacot W, Begbie N, Ke J, Patel G, Curigliano G; DESTINY-Breast06 Trial Investigators. Trastuzumab Deruxtecan after Endocrine Therapy in Metastatic Breast Cancer. N Engl J Med. 2024 Sep 15. doi: 10.1056/NEJMoa2407086. Epub ahead of print. PMID: 39282896.

85. Apolo AB, Ballman KV, Sonpavde G, Berg S, Kim WY, Parikh R, Teo MY, Sweis RF, Geynisman DM, Grivas P, Chatta G, Reichert ZR, Kim JW, Bilen MA, McGregor B, Singh P, Tripathi A, Cole S, Simon N, Niglio S, Ley L, Cordes L, Srinivas S, Huang J, Odegaard M, Watt C, Petrylak D, Hoffman-Censits J, Wen Y, Hahn O, Mitchell C, Tan A, Streicher H, Sharon E, Moon H, Woods M, Halabi S, Perez Burbano G, Morris MJ, Rosenberg JE. Adjuvant Pembrolizumab versus Observation in Muscle-Invasive Urothelial Carcinoma. N Engl J Med. 2024 Sep 15. doi: 10.1056/NEJMoa2401726. Epub ahead of print. PMID: 39282902.

86. Leong T, Smithers BM, Michael M, Haustermans K, Wong R, Gebski V, O'Connell RL, Zalcberg J, Boussioutas A, Findlay M, Willis D, Moore A, Murray WK, Lordick F, O'Callaghan C, Swallow C, Darling G, Miller D, Strickland A, Liberman M, Mineur L, Simes J; Australasian Gastro-Intestinal Trials Group, National Health and Medical Research Council Clinical Trials Centre, Trans-Tasman Radiation Oncology Group, European Organisation for Research and Treatment of Cancer, and Canadian Cancer Trials Group. Preoperative Chemoradiotherapy for Resectable Gastric Cancer. N Engl J Med. 2024 Sep 14. doi: 10.1056/NEJMoa2405195. Epub ahead of print. PMID: 39282905.

87. Wolchok JD, Chiarion-Sileni V, Rutkowski P, Cowey CL, Schadendorf D, Wagstaff J, Queirolo P, Dummer R, Butler MO, Hill AG, Postow MA, Gaudy-Marqueste C, Medina T, Lao CD, Walker J, Márquez-Rodas I, Haanen JBAG, Guidoboni M, Maio M, Schöffski P, Carlino MS, Sandhu S, Lebbé C, Ascierto PA, Long GV, Ritchings C, Nassar A, Askelson M, Benito MP, Wang W, Hodi FS, Larkin J; CheckMate 067 Investigators. Final, 10-Year Outcomes with Nivolumab plus Ipilimumab in Advanced Melanoma. N Engl J Med. 2024 Sep 15. doi: 10.1056/NEJMoa2407417. Epub ahead of print. PMID: 39282897.

88. Hochhaus A, Wang J, Kim DW, Kim DDH, Mayer J, Goh YT, le Coutre P, Takahashi N, Kim I, Etienne G, Andorsky D, Issa GC, Larson RA, Bombaci F, Kapoor S, McCulloch T, Malek K, Yau L, Ifrah S, Hoch M, Cortes JE, Hughes TP; ASC4FIRST Investigators. Asciminib in Newly Diagnosed Chronic Myeloid Leukemia. N Engl J Med. 2024 Sep 12;391(10):885-898. doi: 10.1056/NEJMoa2400858. Epub 2024 May 31. PMID: 38820078.

89. Shuch B et al. [$^{89}$Zr]Zr-girentuximab for PET-CT imaging of clear-cell renal cell carcinoma: A prospective, open-label, multicentre, phase 3 trial. Lancet Oncol 2024 Oct; 25:1277. (https://doi.org/10.1016/S1470-2045(24)00402-9)

90. Hamidi S et al. Initial management of BRAF V600E-variant anaplastic thyroid cancer: The FAST multidisciplinary group consensus statement. JAMA Oncol 2024 Sep 1; 10:1264; [e-pub]. (https://doi.org/10.1001/jamaoncol.2024.2133)

91. Choueiri TK et al. Tivozanib plus nivolumab versus tivozanib monotherapy in patients with renal cell carcinoma following an immune checkpoint inhibitor: Results of the phase 3 TiNivo-2 Study. Lancet 2024 Oct 5; 404:1309. (https://doi.org/10.1016/S0140-6736(24)01758-6)

92. Fan W et al. Survival in patients with recurrent intermediate-stage hepatocellular carcinoma: Sorafenib plus TACE vs TACE alone randomized clinical trial. JAMA Oncol 2024 Aug; 10:1047. (https://doi.org/10.1001/jamaoncol.2024.1831)

93. O'Regan RM et al. Breast cancer index in premenopausal women with early-stage hormone receptor–positive breast cancer. JAMA Oncol 2024 Aug 15; [e-pub]. (https://doi.org/10.1001/jamaoncol.2024.3044)

94. Stout NK et al. Breast cancer screening using mammography, digital breast tomosynthesis, and magnetic resonance imaging by breast density. JAMA Intern Med 2024 Aug 26; [e-pub]. (https://doi.org/10.1001/jamainternmed.2024.4224)

95. de Klaver W et al. Risk of cancers proximal to the colon in fecal immunochemical test positive screenees in a colorectal cancer screening program. Gastroenterology 2024 Sep; 167:788. (https://doi.org/10.1053/j.gastro.2024.04.028)

96. Ohba A et al. Trastuzumab deruxtecan in human epidermal growth factor receptor 2-expressing biliary tract cancer (HERB; NCCH1805): A multicenter, single-arm, phase II trial. J Clin Oncol 2024 Aug 5; JCO2302010; [e-pub]. (https://doi.org/10.1200/JCO.23.02010)

97. Choueiri TK et al. Belzutifan versus everolimus for advanced renal-cell carcinoma. N Engl J Med 2024 Aug 22; 391:710. (https://doi.org/10.1056/NEJMoa2313906)

98. Krämer A et al. Molecularly guided therapy versus chemotherapy after disease control in unfavourable cancer of unknown primary (CUPISCO): An open-label, randomised, phase 2 study. Lancet 2024 Aug 10; 404:527; [e-pub]. (https://doi.org/10.1016/S0140-6736(24)00814-6)

99. Kato K et al. Doublet chemotherapy, triplet chemotherapy, or doublet chemotherapy combined with radiotherapy as neoadjuvant treatment for locally advanced oesophageal cancer (JCOG1109 NExT): A randomised, controlled, open-label, phase 3 trial. Lancet 2024 Jul 6; 404:55. (https://doi.org/10.1016/S0140-6736(24)00745-1)

100. Hamilton MP et al. Risk of second tumors and T-cell lymphoma after CAR T-cell therapy. N Engl J Med 2024 Jun 13; 390:2047. (https://doi.org/10.1056/NEJMoa2401361)

101. Ozdemirli M et al. Indolent CD4+ CAR T-cell lymphoma after cilta-cel CAR-T cell therapy. N Engl J Med 2024 Jun 13; 390:2074. (https://doi.org/10.1056/NEJMoa2401530)

102. Mitchell E and Vassiliou GS. T-cell cancer after CAR T-cell therapy. N Engl J Med 2024 Jun 13; 390:2120. (https://doi.org/10.1056/NEJMe2405538)

103. Facon T et al. Isatuximab, bortezomib, lenalidomide, and dexamethasone for multiple myeloma. N Engl J Med 2024 Jun 3; [e-pub]. (https://doi.org/10.1056/NEJMoa2400712)

104. Liu X et al. Induction-concurrent chemoradiotherapy with or without sintilimab in patients with locoregionally advanced nasopharyngeal carcinoma in China (CONTINUUM): A multicentre, open-label, parallel-group, randomised, controlled, phase 3 trial. Lancet 2024 Jun 22; 403:2720. (https://doi.org/10.1016/S0140-6736(24)00594-4)

105. van As N, Griffin C, Tree A, Patel J, Ostler P, van der Voet H, Loblaw A, Chu W, Ford D, Tolan S, Jain S, Camilleri P, Kancherla K, Frew J, Chan A, Naismith O, Armstrong J, Staffurth J, Martin A, Dayes I, Wells P, Price D, Williamson E, Pugh J, Manning G, Brown S, Burnett S, Hall E. Phase 3 Trial of Stereotactic Body Radiotherapy in Localized Prostate Cancer. N Engl J Med. 2024 Oct 17;391(15):1413-1425. doi: 10.1056/NEJMoa2403365. PMID: 39413377; PMCID: PMC7616714.

106. Hu JC, Assel M, Allaf ME, Vickers AJ, Ehdaie B, Cohen AJ, Green DA, Ghazi A, Ristau BT, Kowalczyk KJ, George AK, Patel HD, Montgomery JS, Han M, Rezaee M, Pavlovich CP, Patel NA, Ross AE, Kundu SD, Wang GJ, Shoag JE, Singla N, Stensland K, Gorin MA, Schaeffer AJ, Schaeffer EM. Transperineal vs Transrectal Prostate Biopsy-The PREVENT Randomized Clinical Trial. JAMA Oncol. 2024 Sep 19:e244000. doi: 10.1001/jamaoncol.2024.4000. Epub ahead of print. PMID: 39298143; PMCID: PMC11413751.

107. Morris MJ et al. 177Lu-PSMA-617 versus a change of androgen receptor pathway inhibitor therapy for taxane-naive patients with progressive metastatic castration-resistant prostate cancer (PSMAfore): A phase 3, randomised, controlled trial. Lancet 2024 Sep 15; [e-pub]. (https://doi.org/10.1016/S0140-6736(24)01653-2)

108. Della Porta MG et al. Luspatercept versus epoetin alfa in erythropoiesis-stimulating agent-naive, transfusion-dependent, lower-risk myelodysplastic syndromes (COMMANDS): Primary analysis of a phase 3, open-label, randomised, controlled trial. Lancet Haematology 2024 Sep; 11:e646. (https://doi.org/10.1016/S2352-3026(24)00203-5109.

109. Potter AL et al. Pack-year smoking history: An inadequate and biased measure to determine lung cancer screening eligibility. J Clin Oncol 2024 Jun 10; 42:2026. (https://doi.org/10.1200/JCO.23.01780)

110. Gallois C et al. Oxaliplatin-based adjuvant chemotherapy in older patients with stage III colon cancer: An ACCENT/IDEA pooled analysis of 12 trials. J Clin Oncol 2024 Mar 28; [e-pub]. (https://doi.org/10.1200/JCO.23.01326)

111. Shitara K et al. Neoadjuvant and adjuvant pembrolizumab plus chemotherapy in locally advanced gastric or gastro-oesophageal cancer (KEYNOTE-585): An interim analysis of the multicentre, double-blind, randomised phase 3 study. Lancet Oncol 2023 Dec 19; [e-pub]. (https://doi.org/10.1016/S1470-2045(23)00541-7)

112. Dimopoulos MA, Beksac M, Pour L, Delimpasi S, Vorobyev V, Quach H, Spicka I, Radocha J, Robak P, Kim K, Cavo M, Suzuki K, Morris K, Pompilus F, Phillips-Jones A, Zhou XL, Fulci G, Sule N, Kremer BE, Opalinska J, Mateos MV, Trudel S; DREAMM-8 Investigators. Belantamab Mafodotin, Pomalidomide, and Dexamethasone in Multiple Myeloma. N Engl J Med. 2024 Aug 1;391(5):408-421. doi: 10.1056/NEJMoa2403407. Epub 2024 Jun 2. PMID: 38828951.

Made in the USA
Monee, IL
05 November 2026

67383552R00064